Ending the ECZEMA EPIDEMIC

Ending the ECZEMA EPIDEMIC

Surprising Solutions to Transform
Your Child's Skin from Within

Featuring The Eczema Kitchen by Lindsay Kingdon

Ana-Maria Temple, MD & John Temple, MD

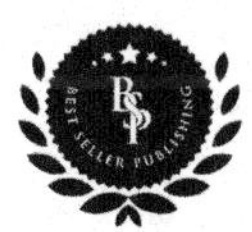

Published by Best Seller Publishing®, St. Augustine, FL
Best Seller Publishing® is a registered trademark.
Printed in the United States of America.

ISBN:978-1959840404

For more information, please write:
Best Seller Publishing®
53 Marine Street
St. Augustine, FL 32084
or call 1 (626) 765-9750
Visit us online at: www.BestSellerPublishing.org

Praise for The Eczema Transformation Program

"When Vivienne was three months old, we were told by her dermatologist that her severe eczema could be a lifelong, mysterious, and chronic condition. Six months later, after being in the course for several months, her skin became soft, porcelain, mostly itch- and flare-free. We stay on top of her skin care routine, diet, supplements, and do still use topicals in small areas. We are blown away (her doctors are, too) at the progress she's made. Thank you SO MUCH, Ana-Maria Temple and team, for all that you do. My eyes get full when I think about HOW grateful our entire family is for the wisdom you share and all the work you are doing to heal kids from the inside out."

Alexandra

"Our son was covered, head to toe. We had spent $25,000 on doctors, even going out of state many times. No one cared and everyone's answer was *steroids*. When I came to you, Dr. Temple, Mattis had it all over his face and his entire body. We never slept, we never had peace. Our son couldn't function. I wanted to tell you that our son is now clear. He is thriving in preschool and catching up to his peers. I'm so thankful we found you, and I will be putting a package together to give other moms with your information as well as foods we ate, etc. Please know how big of a life change this was. We prayed hard for two years and God brought us to you. In less than six months Mattis is clear!! Thank you for everything."

Rachel

"It works ... it's not always linear, it's such hard work, and some days it seems like nothing is happening. But we've gone from having to watch every single (limited) thing that went in my daughter's mouth to being able to expand her menu so much. And most importantly, she's not miserable scratching and fussing anymore. So thankful!"

Neely

"I have to tell you, our lives have been changed by this program! I fully believe in it and I have been telling everyone I know about the changes I've seen in my family, not just my son's skin.

Behavior, ability to learn and participate at school, sleep habits, and of course the poops! It has impacted everything we do and our outlook on life and health. And the funny thing is, all the things you preach should be obvious ... but they aren't! Despite the many, many specialists we have seen, not one of them suggested eliminating the most basic, scientifically proven irritants like sugar, dyes, and preservatives. I hate to think of where we would be without this program."

Grace

"I've had seasonal allergies and mild asthma since I was a kid. I grew up in a conventional farm family, so I've been around chemicals most of my life. My asthma and allergies started to get worse as an adult. When we were pregnant with our oldest, I started questioning the chemicals I was using and started learning more about the crops I was growing. I left my family's conventional farm and started transitioning my acres to organic in 2016. Thus, it really wasn't hard for me to get on board when Megan joined Dr. Temple's eczema course for our kids. I wasn't overly excited to give up my ice cream, but I knew I had to as an example to our children. I wasn't expecting my asthma and allergies to disappear, almost completely, only weeks after removing gluten and dairy from my diet. The results are hard to ignore. We've also been very pleased with the results we've seen in our children. My two-and-a-half-year-old doesn't have itchy skin anymore, and my sixteen-month-old son's bumps on his thighs and arms have started to fade. Thank you for this program and for all the support you've provided our family."

Jeff Janes

"THANK YOU, THANK YOU, THANK YOU!! I seriously cannot say it enough! Dr. T and Lindsay have changed our lives. At 2 months old, my daughter was covered in eczema head to toe. She scratched 24/7, and neither of us got any sleep. She dropped from the 40th percentile in all measurements down to less than 1. After just a couple months on this course her eczema was nearly gone, and now at seven months in she only has occasional, mild patches on her hands and feet. She's back up to the 17th percentile in weight and height, and in the 90th for her head! She sleeps through the night. She can ride in the car with no mittens (I truly never thought I'd see the day). She can wear shorts and short sleeves without scratching until she bleeds. She has also "outgrown" two food allergies and her dog allergy, and is close to outgrowing a third food allergy. To say you turned our lives around is an understatement. I truly don't know where we would be without you. This course is worth every penny and then some. If I would've known about this when she first developed eczema it would have saved me thousands of dollars. I cannot endorse this program enough! I want to fly to NC to hug you two!"

Tiffany Williams

"The eczema course has truly changed our lives and has taught us so much. Both of our children suffered from eczema, other random skin rashes, and digestive problems. After we decided to try strictly eliminating gluten and dairy, we saw great improvement but still continued to have issues as time went on. The course filled in the missing pieces for us. Our children's skin has completely cleared up and their digestion has normalized. We have also come to realize that issues with poor sleep and irritability were also related. Overall mood has greatly improved and they are both sleeping like champs.

"In addition, my husband suffered from severe seasonal allergies and frequent debilitating migraines for years. I was diagnosed with two different skin conditions, which were unsuccessfully treated with prescription creams. Once we joined the program for our children and applied the lessons to our lives, our symptoms almost disappeared completely without the need for medication.

"Dr. Temple and Lindsay are both a wealth of knowledge. Since beginning the course, they have always answered all of my questions and have helped me to tweak things as needed to individualize the program to our needs and help us achieve success. I highly recommend this program. It has been worth every penny! Thank you so much Dr. Temple and Lindsay!"

Jackie

"I wanted to let everyone know how helpful and really a lifesaver this program has been for me and my son. Isaac is twenty months now and is doing so much better than when we started some months ago. We still have challenges, but I so appreciate Dr. Temple and Lindsay because I know I have a place to go, and I do not feel so alone. Parenting a child with eczema is heart-wrenching, and I thank Dr. Temple and Lindsay from the bottom of my heart, not only for their sound and practical advice, but also for offering what we need most, hope and patience. I'm so grateful that Dr. Temple is whip-smart and yet she is open and listens, so very different than other doctors that offered horrible advice and made me feel like my instincts do not matter. Eczema transformation is a better way, so much better."

Sonya

Contents

Introduction

Why Me?

I remember sitting in a doctor's office in the spring of 2007 with my three sick kids, feeling hopeless. I was utterly confused, frustrated, and alone. They were 2, 4, and 6 years old. All three were battling chronic disease, such as eczema, asthma, constipation, severe seasonal allergies, recurrent ear infections, recurrent croup, and behavioral issues. I was a pediatrician, five years in practice, and had zero answers aside from prescribing steroids, antibiotics, antihistamines, and laxatives. How could this be?

In 1995, I attended one of the best medical schools in the country, where I learned that, in the United States, we supposedly have the best medical care and the latest advances for treating disease. Despite those advances, I stared in disbelief at yet more prescription medications for the tiny humans in front of me. I thought, *Are these the only options for my ill children?* I refused to believe this. I knew something had to change. My mind started buzzing. I thought, *If the medicines prescribed were doing their job, why were my kids getting sicker and sicker and never getting better? Why does eczema keep coming back?*

You know that moment when the Mama Warrior arrives? She appears the day our children are born and is always there in the background—but one day, she takes over our body, soul, and mind, and it's on!

It was on that day, in that sterile doctor's office in April 2007, with my three little ducklings looking up at me begging for relief, that Mama Warrior took over and said, *This will not be my children's story. I refuse to believe that medications, lotions, and specialist visits are the answer to their issues. There is more to this tale, and we are just not digging deep enough.*

Truth be told, I had no idea what the heck she was going to do, but I had a vision: my children would be able to sleep without scratching; their arms and legs would stop bleeding; colds would no longer turn into ear infections or croup; snot would no longer be the norm in the household; and packing for travel would no longer include prescription lotions and medications. The children would roll in the grass without bursting into hives, go on Easter egg hunts without their eyes swelling shut, and visit friends and relatives without scratching. They would run, play, and laugh, and medications would be a thing of the past. It would be an inspirational story to tell others.

A few days later, I went to a nutrition talk at my children's elementary school. At 7:30 in the morning, sitting in a first grader's chair with my knees to my chest and freezing to death from the blasting air conditioning, I heard the speaker say, "Are you feeding your children this?" as she pointed to sugar-loaded snacks like Go-GURTS, chocolate milk, and Uncrustables. The first step in my children's journey materialized. Sugar. A piece of the puzzle appeared, and I had my first step toward wellness outlined.

And that is how we started. I took an inventory of the amount of sugar in my children's diet and, frankly, I was appalled. I then took a look at food coloring and I learned about ingredients, micronutrients, and so on. Slowly, over the next five years, my children stopped needing antibiotics, creams, steroids, and doctor visits. One step led to another, and the kids got better. They thrived without coughing, scratching, itching, or bleeding.

In the meantime, my dog, a giant and handsome Rhodesian Ridgeback, developed weird skin lesions on several occasions. When I took him to the vet for the third time, the doctor explained, "This is a common skin issue with this breed, and he just needs another course of steroids and antibiotics." Really? Here we go again. Having learned from my kids' healing journey, I turned my attention to the dog's food and added the kids' supplements (vitamin D and omega-3 fatty acids) in giant dog doses. Low and behold, his coat improved and he became even more handsome. The skin issues never recurred.

Speaking of handsome, my husband battled chronic urticaria (hives) and seasonal allergies for most of his life. Of note—he was not on board with all the "voodoo" stuff I was doing for the kids. In fact, we fought over it for five years. He was upset I threw his favorite sugary cereals and Cheez-Its crackers in the trash. He would also come home from work and exclaim in frustration, "Why is our grocery bill so high?"

As you will learn later, he finally had his *Aha* moment and began to shift his mindset. The hives went away, his joints stopped hurting, and his seasonal allergies improved significantly. Once he saw the results, he became so inspired that now he is my co-author on this book. Yes, folks, we can change our eating and lifestyle habits at forty years old.

Why You?

Have you ...

- Sat in your pediatrician's office wondering if steroids should be the first line of treatment for your child's skin condition?
- Felt helpless as you watched your child itch and bleed?
- Wondered why your child's eczema keeps getting worse?
- Googled for hours on end, searching for creams and spending a lot of money without getting any results?
- Questioned why, despite cleaning up their diet, your children still have eczema?
- Pondered why a baby who is breastfed only has developed eczema?

Why This Topic?

If you or your child is suffering from eczema, take solace in the notion that you are not alone.

Eczema (also known as atopic dermatitis) is the body's way of letting us know something is amiss on the inside. It is not simply an annoying skin condition. As you will learn in this book, eczema is a sign of total body inflammation and if ignored, or treated with topical approaches only, it will progress to other diseases.

- 80% of kids with eczema develop hay fever or asthma later in childhood.[1]
- 50% of children with severe eczema will develop asthma.[2]
- 30% of children with eczema develop a food allergy.[3]

---

1 https://acaai.org/allergies/allergic-conditions/skin-allergy/eczema/

2 https://pubmed.ncbi.nlm.nih.gov/17655920/

3 https://pubmed.ncbi.nlm.nih.gov/26897122/

- 6% of kids with eczema develop ADHD.[4]
- Children and adolescents with eczema are two to six times more likely to have depression, anxiety, or a conduct disorder than children without eczema.[5]
- Teens and adults with eczema are up to 44% more likely to exhibit suicidal ideation, and 36% more likely to attempt suicide.[6]
- 20% of children with eczema will continue to have this issue in adulthood.[7]

Why My Approach?

I know you are busy and overwhelmed with your child's eczema and all the information coming at you from all sorts of places. That's why this book is different. After twenty years of treating eczema, I have seen the problem from almost every angle. The families I have treated along the way, including my own, hold fascinating stories and clues to a better way to manage eczema. I start each chapter with my real-life encounters, which many of you will, no doubt, identify with. Within these stories I outline treatment plans and takeaways parents and caregivers can implement right away.

One of the overarching themes after so many years of meeting families with eczema is the amount of misconception and misinformation out there about the disease. Thus, an appropriate place to start is squashing some of the most common misconceptions I have encountered.

---

[4] https://pubmed.ncbi.nlm.nih.gov/23245818/
[5] https://pubmed.ncbi.nlm.nih.gov/23245818/
[6] https://pubmed.ncbi.nlm.nih.gov/30365995/
[7] https://pubmed.ncbi.nlm.nih.gov/27544489/

1

Eczema Misconceptions

Before we delve into the nitty-gritty of eczema, I think it's appropriate to address some of the elephants in the room (fun fact: some countries have unsuccessfully used elephant skin to treat eczema!). The elephants in the room are the alarming number of myths and misconceptions that surround eczema and its treatment. I can tell you that these misconceptions are firmly rooted in the minds of Americans because they nearly ended my marriage.

My husband, John, and I met at the University of North Carolina at Chapel Hill School of Medicine, a traditional Western medical school. Neither of us had any exposure to functional medicine or holistic practice during our time there, and our education around nutrition was sorely lacking. As we both began our practices, we fell into the standard 10-minute appointments and a prescription given on the way out the door. But the day I realized my own children's sickness was largely related to our diet, everything changed—including my marriage.

That day, more than ten years ago, remains vivid in my mind. I walked into our pantry with a large industrial trash can and began the clean-out. Frosted Flakes, Cinnamon Toast Crunch, and Honey Bunches of Oats boxes were flying through the air, while the Goldfish crackers, Cheez-Its crackers, and Pringles potato chips followed. I worked my way to the refrigerator and freezer, removing chicken nuggets, Uncrustables, frozen burritos, pizzas, Go-GURTS, and juice boxes. It was such a catharsis, throwing these symbols of my children's sickness away. But it was not without consequences.

John walked in from a long day at work and wandered into the pantry for his daily fix of sugary cereal. I sat bracing myself for the storm that was brewing in our kitchen. "Ana-Maria! What the #$@!% happened in the pantry?" he shouted. "Where is the cereal?"

I calmly explained to him that the sugar-laden food in our pantry was harming our family. He blew up. "What are you talking about? No one in our family is overweight! Sugar has nothing to do with allergies and eczema!"

I stuck to my guns and responded, "I went to a nutritionist's presentation at the kids' school, and the speaker explained the connection between food and childhood illness, with one of the biggest culprits being sugar."

The battle ensued for 30 minutes that day and for five years of our marriage. When I began buying only organic food to avoid the toxic pesticides that can worsen eczema, John was sitting at home with the grocery bill and a scowl on his face. He actually compared our previous bills to the current ones with healthier options, which over the course of a few months, cost a few hundred dollars more. It was not that much in the big scheme of things (just look at your cell phone bills, cable bills, and the cost of eating out), but John just didn't see the value.

When we would go to dinner and I would inquire about certain ingredients in the food I was ordering, John was mortified. He said we were becoming like "those tree-hugging people" who are crazy about food, only eat kale and carrots, and are basically conspiracy theorists. He pointed to professional athletes he worshipped, like Michael Jordan, who only seemed to eat at McDonald's (according to the commercials) yet were in amazing physical condition.

If you look at popular culture, you can see John's point—we embrace overindulgence, supersizing, and a "spend now, pay later" attitude. We both grew up inundated with food commercials for Cocoa Pops, Fruity Pebbles, McDonald's, and frozen pizzas—heat-and-eat meals made for convenience, not nutrition.

We both operated under the assumption that overindulgence in food leads to obesity, but we believed the lie that food quality is unrelated to disease. Basically, we believed food *quantity* was the key factor rather than food *quality*. I was forced to look at it in a different way when my children's health continued to deteriorate, despite all my efforts. But John was a much slower convert, as are many husbands whom I meet.

My experience is that men tend to have a strong cognitive bias about food. Cognitive bias is a blind spot or a limitation in thought, and it's caused by the tendency of our brain to perceive information through a filter of personal experiences and preferences. Thus, men will tend to say, "I ate this as a kid and I am fine!" allowing them to disregard new information about a food's quality. I find that many of the misconceptions about eczema tend to stem from a cognitive bias set forth by the traditional medical system. Despite taking the Hippocratic oath, traditional medical doctors seemed to have forgotten Hippocrates' other sage advice: "Let thy food be thy medicine, and medicine be thy food." Nowadays, it can be hard to judge which is more toxic, our diets or all the medications we take.

Americans tend to think that all diseases are best treated with a pill. Hence, we have the highest usage of prescription medication in the world. However, our country's overall health does not even rank in the top 20 worldwide (the average American takes four prescription pills per day and even more supplements).[8] And for kids under the age of 12, nearly 20 percent have taken a prescription drug every month. And it gets even more abysmal the older you get: 27 percent of adolescents aged 12–19, 46.7 percent of adults aged 20–59, and 85 percent of adults aged 60+ used prescription drugs every month.[9]

In our situation, John simply did not see the value in dietary change because none of us were overweight. The interesting (frustrating) thing about his bias about food is that he was meticulous about quality in so many other areas of his life. He would only put high-octane, premium gas in his new car, he would only purchase products recommended by Consumer Reports, and he was fanatical about clothing material and quality. But nowhere along the way did the concept of sugar or food chemicals that caused disease take hold. Thus began years of friction over this issue and a major divide in our household.

John would continue to buy and eat highly processed, sugary foods in front of our children, who couldn't understand why they were being excluded from such yumminess. In fact, he would have an industrial-sized box of Cheez-Its next to his chair each night at dinner to complement his meal, while the kids begged for one. You can imagine my struggles to introduce whole foods and vegetables to my kids, while my husband dished out highly addictive crackers at dinner.

Have you ever been in a situation with your family where you knew in your heart that something was wrong, but you and your partner simply could not agree? Or even more commonly, you and your spouse disagree on how to manage a basic problem

---

8 https://worldpopulationreview.com/country-rankings/healthiest-countries

9 https://www.cdc.gov/nchs/products/databriefs/db334.htm

with your kids? I would have never thought that one of the biggest issues in my marriage would surround food, but I guess I have learned never to say never in a marriage.

This is why I want to start by addressing misconceptions about eczema. Sometimes our assumptions about a problem are so deeply rooted that we can't even imagine another way. In retrospect, there were probably more constructive and less confrontational ways to broach this subject with John all those years ago.

Sometimes just asking the following question can disarm a strong cognitive bias: "I understand that this new way of thinking sounds foreign to you, but are you willing to think about it from a different perspective for the sake of our kids?"

As you read through the following common misconceptions about eczema, ask yourself the question above. Are you open to thinking about eczema in a whole new way? We will dissect each of these in upcoming chapters, but now is the time to start placing those preconceived notions aside.

Deep, Deep Roots: Seven Common Misconceptions About Eczema

1. Eczema is a skin disease

Eczema appears on the skin; thus, it is reasonable to believe that it is an isolated skin problem. But our skin is simply a window into our gut, and when our skin isn't happy, neither is our gut. I believe eczema is nature's way of telling us there is a problem inside. Treating eczema is about healing from the inside out. Pharmaceutical companies want you to believe the opposite, because the average cost to initiate advanced therapy for severe eczema is $20,722.[10] Additionally, more than half of families with eczema spend more than $1,000 per year on eczema treatments.[11] If families were to reduce the eczema burden by healing their guts, Big Pharma would lose billions. When we treat only the symptoms of a disease, we become a customer for life. When we address the runaway immune system that is central to ending the Eczema Epidemic, we allow long-term healing to occur.

2. Eczema is curable/incurable

First, I think it's important to differentiate *healing* from *curing*. Curing implies someone or something else has eradicated the disease—like a pill, for example. Americans have been taught that a "cure" for any disease is always one treatment away. Healing implies that your body has done the work of limiting the disease and restoring balance. When we break a bone and it heals, we are not cured—the bone will never be the same again. But the bone is remodeled and function is restored. Our skin works in much the same way. When we cut ourselves or get sunburned, the body reliably puts the skin-repair cells to work to bridge the broken skin or slough the damaged layer. Though we are sometimes left with a scar, function has been restored and the skin is healed. I believe if we correct and optimize our immune systems, we will allow our bodies to "heal" eczema.

3. You can resolve eczema with diet alone

Although food is often implicated in the development of eczema, it is not the only factor. The origins of eczema are complex and multifaceted. Thus, we must approach the treatment from many angles, such as environmental factors like cleaners and toxic chemicals, stress, histamines, parental factors, vitamin and

---

[10] https://www.ncbi.nlm.nih.gov/pmc/articles/PMC7367964/

[11] https://pubmed.ncbi.nlm.nih.gov/33323748/

mineral deficiencies, skin and gut microbiome considerations, and much more.

Patients and families who see me in the office or join one of my online eczema programs often say, "We have already tried everything and it's not getting better." Usually, they mean they have tried some dietary changes and creams, but I find most have not taken a holistic approach to eczema. Remember, a holistic approach is characterized by the treatment of the whole person, not just one organ. It means taking into account the person, family, community, and culture, as well as environmental, mental, and social factors, rather than just the symptoms of a disease.

4. If you could just find that *one thing*, the eczema would resolve

Eczema creams, topicals, and medications make up a billion-dollar industry. Companies are banking on you trying dozens of products to find "the one" miracle cure. Remember the old saying, "If it seems too good to be true, it probably is"? Unfortunately, healing eczema typically means making some hard lifestyle changes and acknowledging that the big, red "Easy" button doesn't exist.

Eczema typically takes months or even years to develop, and it can take just as long to address the root causes. Many families jump from one treatment to the next in the hope of finding a silver bullet and quickly become frustrated when the results don't progress quickly. For example, if one has cancer, or a weight problem, people generally understand that it will take months, if not years, to get better. But when it comes to eczema—where a steroid cream (which is little more than a Band-Aid) can make the symptoms go away in 24 hours—most people have developed the perception that this chronic disease should get better in one day.

5. Genetics determine who will develop eczema

Many families believe that eczema is in their genes, and therefore they have no control over its development. I could NOT disagree more—genetics may load the gun, but our environment, lifestyle, diet, and stress pull the trigger. The entire field of epigenetics has shown us that genes are NOT the sole determinant of disease, but just one factor in the ultimate development of diseases. It's in our power to alter the way our genes are expressed, which in turn lessens our risk of chronic disease.

It's in our power to alter the way our genes are expressed, which in turn lessens our risk of chronic disease.

6. Kids will outgrow eczema

Many parents assume eczema is like diaper rash or teething, and that, with time, it will resolve on its own. The reality is that 10–30 percent of kids will have eczema that lasts well into adulthood.[12] In fact, every American adult has a 1 in 10 chance of developing eczema in their lifetime.[13] Eczema is an external sign of other issues lurking below the surface. We must start the process of root cause analysis to find out why it has started in a child or even in an adult, because the eczema might appear to be resolved, but other things such as seasonal allergies, asthma, anxiety, or ADHD will appear. To a lot of people, it may seem that these are all just different, unrelated things. However, if we look at these chronic diseases as rooted in inflammation that starts in the gut, we can start to see that eczema is more like a warning sign from the body of things to come.

---

[12] https://pubmed.ncbi.nlm.nih.gov/24696036/

[13] https://www.ncbi.nlm.nih.gov/pmc/articles/PMC4349386/

7. Eczema typically begins at the age of 3–6 months

Although the first physical signs of eczema may not appear until the first few months of life, the disease process has usually started before birth. Various pre-birth factors—such as maternal diet, maternal stress, maternal and paternal microbiomes, birth method (C-section versus vaginal), and medications during pregnancy and delivery—all play a role in eczema development.

Additionally, parental factors beyond genetics play a role in passing on eczema risk. Remember, a newborn develops most of its microbiome based on the parents' microbiomes. So, if mom and dad had sick guts before birth, this will be ultimately passed on to the baby.

Cracker Sacrifice

I desperately wish John had had a book like this to read ten years ago, when we started this journey. With each passing day, I held my ground on my children's diet but respected John's opinions. We had reached something of a stalemate. Then something transformational happened to John—he started getting sicker. He had worsening GI symptoms after those bowls of cereal, more aches and pains in his joints, frequent colds, and then pneumonia. He was working 80-hour weeks building a surgery practice, often late into the night. One morning he simply could not get out of bed. I was worried, since this was a guy who would puke in trash cans between surgeries (or even during) but never cancel the five remaining surgeries that day.

Then he started coughing up blood but didn't want to go to the hospital—once again proving that doctors are horrible patients. We were supposed to leave on a long-awaited trip to Paris in a few days, and there was no way I was going to let this stubborn lug spoil our trip. I dragged him from the bed to the emergency room. A chest X-ray revealed double pneumonia. Although it took him days to get out of bed, when he woke up, he also did so symbolically. He began to question his lifestyle and choices. He began to accept the fact that his diet might be a problem. (Progress is slow, people.)

Nonetheless, he knew something was wrong and agreed to try my approach. He started slowly at first—just giving up his beloved Cheez-Its. Then, he gave up fast food. Finally, he stopped the cereal, and that was a game changer. Joint aches resolved and he had no more colds. Once he had a few victories, all the dominoes fell. Not only did John change his diet, he also transformed his life. But the biggest change in John was his mindset—and changing your mindset is really the key to beginning your eczema healing journey.

A fascinating study on milkshakes reinforces the importance of mindset in changing our bodies.[14] Participants were given the impression that the researchers were studying the physiological effects of milkshakes with "vastly different" amounts of nutrients, fats, and calories. Subjects were told the research was being done to potentially help hospital patients with different needs for calories or nutrients. The participants would drink the shake, and then researchers would measure the physiological response in their bodies via blood tests.

Researchers were primarily looking at blood levels of the hormone ghrelin, also known as the hunger hormone. Basically, when you are feeling hungry, ghrelin levels go up; when you are full, ghrelin levels go down. By measuring this, researchers could tell how filling each milkshake really was. The participants were told they would try two different shakes on two different occasions. They were told the first shake was packed with calories

[14] https://pubmed.ncbi.nlm.nih.gov/21574706/

and nutrients and contained more than 620 calories (this was called the "indulgent mindset" shake). They were told the second shake was much lighter, containing only 140 calories with fewer ingredients (this was called the "sensible mindset" shake). But here's the catch—*they all were drinking the exact same shake!*

The mindset of indulgence produced a dramatically steeper decline in ghrelin after consuming the shake, whereas the mindset of sensibility produced a relatively flat ghrelin response. Participants' physiological response to the shake *was shaped more by what they believed* they were drinking than by the actual nutritional value of the shake they drank. WOW!

New Beginnings

John ultimately left his lucrative surgical career after years of frustration with the traditional Western system. "I simply believed less and less in the procedures I was performing," John said, while reflecting on his career change. He found that the orthopedic community failed to treat the person as a whole and just focused on body parts. That knee joint is connected to a person, and if you don't treat the whole person, your knee procedure is likely to fail. The atmosphere in his orthopedic practice just couldn't accommodate that type of holistic approach—neither, it seems, can many medical groups around the country.

This was my same feeling when I left my busy pediatrics practice in 2017 to open a holistic clinic. As our visions have aligned over the past few years, John and I have learned to collaborate toward common goals of overall community wellness.

Although we still occasionally disagree on certain medical topics, the nature of our debates has drastically changed. We now approach disagreements seeking to find out what the other person knows, rather than attempting to convince them our side is right. After all, everyone you will ever meet knows something you don't.

Now that we have all agreed to approach eczema with open hearts and minds, let's move on to a very divisive topic—allergy and food testing.

Chapter Takeaways

- We need to change our mindset around how we approach disease in the Western world, acknowledging the cognitive biases we bring to the eczema diagnosis.
- Eczema is a complex, multifaceted disease, with rampant misinformation circulating regarding its origins and treatments.
- Altering my own family's diet and lifestyle to manage eczema not only healed my children's skin, it fundamentally changed our lives.

For more information about food allergy testing or our Eczema Transformation Program, please visit the book resource page by scanning the QR code below.

2

Allergens Versus Intolerance/Sensitivity

My family has dealt with eczema for nearly twenty years. My middle child, Jake, had his most severe symptoms during middle school and high school. He never had any type of severe reaction to food, like a peanut allergy for instance, so we assumed his skin problems were NOT food-related. We noticed he didn't like to take his shirt off at the pool, as he became more self-conscious over the appearance of his skin. He had large areas of red, inflamed eczema patches on his chest that would routinely bleed after scratching. Despite topical steroids (started before I realized the error of my ways), his symptoms continued to worsen, particularly on his chest, back, and face.

Jake has always been my best eater and preferred the "anything" diet—meaning you could put just about anything in front of him and he would eat it. This is great when you introduce a child to new whole foods, fruits, and vegetables, but it's a curse at birthday parties, restaurants, and buffets. When Jake was old enough to have a mature discussion over his skin, I was able to convince him that his food choices were likely playing a role in his eczema. Even though we had cleaned up things like sugars and processed foods, the crusty bleeding areas persisted on his chest and back.

He told me, "Mom, I hate that I'm the only kid at the pool who doesn't take their shirt off because I don't want the kids to make fun of my skin. I will do whatever it takes to make the eczema go away." I was inspired yet heartbroken for him at the same time. It's miserable to watch your children suffer, and I felt responsible. I had tried some elimination diets with Jake in the past, but it was still difficult for me to determine what his food triggers were.

I had just transitioned to my holistic practice and discovered a different type of food test that checks the blood for a more subtle type of reaction. My training had taught me that traditional skin testing was the only option to evaluate for a food allergy, but I subsequently learned that food allergies and sensitivities were much more complex. I also was concerned that Jake would start to eliminate too many foods from his diet because he was so impacted by the social implications of his eczema. With this in mind, I sent Jake for this newer food test, which uses a blood test rather than classic skin testing. We will explore the details of this newer food test later in the chapter.

If the world of food allergy testing was this complex to me, I can't imagine how a non-medical parent must feel when navigating this process. Have you ever felt like you were drowning in information and opinions while your child was in crisis? The holistic and traditional medical communities cannot agree on the best way forward for testing food allergies and sensitivities in children, and unfortunately, families suffer. I continue to get so many questions on the difference between food allergies, sensitivities, and intolerance that I feel we should address this early in the book to give you a baseline understanding.

The three primary terms used when discussing issues with food are *food allergy*, *food sensitivity*, and *food intolerance*. These terms get thrown around so much that the differences between them have been blurred over time, leading to appropriate skepticism from critics. I think it's important to understand each term and how it was originally intended to describe issues with food.

Defining the Term *Food Allergy*

Food allergy describes an acute immune reaction to a protein in certain foods. Most people have a general understanding of allergies to foods such as peanuts, tree nuts, cow's milk, eggs, soy, wheat, seafood, or shellfish. I even had a friend who swore he was deathly allergic to bananas. Western medicine fully accepts the concept of food allergies and typically supports testing for them. Food allergies cause such an immediate and severe immune inflammatory response that they can be life-threatening.

You have probably heard of someone with a peanut allergy who, upon exposure to peanuts, may have difficulty breathing, acute hives, and a racing heart rate, and who may die if not urgently treated. In fact, many define their allergy by how much time they have to access their EpiPen before their airway closes. To understand this type of immune response, we must first learn a bit about the immune system in general.

We have cells in our body that float around in our blood, feeling everything they pass. When they feel something that is foreign and that they perceive as dangerous, they begin a cascade of events to protect the body from the invader. One of those events is remembering the shape of the invader they just encountered and manufacturing antibodies against it for future defense. That's why you must first be exposed to a virus or food that causes your body to make antibodies, so that in subsequent exposures, your body is ready to react. (This is why no rash occurs when you touch poison ivy for the first time in your life—but the next time, watch out!)

Sometimes, the body mistakenly makes antibodies against molecules that are actually friendly components of the food we eat or even a part of the body itself. (This is the concept behind autoimmune disease.) The higher the inflammatory state the body is in, the more likely it is to create antibodies against friendly things. This is why some people tend to have multiple allergies.

> **The higher the inflammatory state the body is in, the more likely it is to create antibodies against friendly things. This is why some people tend to have multiple allergies.**

Our bodies create different types of antibodies based on how severe and acute it perceives the threat to be. This makes sense from an evolutionary standpoint because something that's poisonous could kill us quickly; it thus requires a more immediate response than a cold or virus that is not as acute a threat. The body puts acute food allergy into the highest threat category and creates an antibody (Ab) known as immunoglobulin E (IgE). When the IgE system gets activated, the body mounts an overly aggressive response that can be life-threatening.

This response is so sensitive that you can typically test for it just by placing the problem substance on the skin. This is the idea behind the most standardized type of food allergy test: skin testing. Dozens of substances are tested by placing small amounts on a patient's back, one at a time, and waiting to see if any of them cause an acute skin reaction. Western medicine has traditionally taught (incorrectly) that if you don't have an acute skin response, then you have no issue with that particular food.

However, there are several problems with this approach. First, skin testing has only been shown to be about 85 percent accurate in detecting these allergies. This means that 15 percent of patients will have an acute food allergy that doesn't show up on testing but may be wreaking havoc on the immune system. The second issue is that we now believe that certain foods may stimulate another part of the immune system that is more subtle in its reaction. This other side of the immune system is where we believe much of the connection exists between eczema and food. Because the massive, acute allergic response does not occur with these foods, it has been termed *food sensitivity*.

Defining *Food Sensitivity*

As described above, the body creates different types of antibodies based on how severe it deems the threat from a particular foreign substance. If the body created IgE antibodies for every foreign substance, we would constantly be faced with life-threatening immune responses for things that aren't all that dangerous. So, the body has other types of antibodies to deal with these less acute situations. The one we will focus on for eczema is called immunoglobulin G (IgG).

IgG is created for long-term defense against foreign invaders. For example, when we become immune to chickenpox after having had the disease, it is the IgG antibodies that are providing that immunity. Over the past twenty years, compelling evidence has emerged that a number of chronic diseases may be related to food and an IgG antibody response to that food. While an IgE antibody allergic response occurs between seconds and minutes, IgG antibody response takes anywhere from hours to a week. Thus, they are very difficult to find by skin testing. You can use a blood test to find IgG antibodies to many foods, but this is where the major controversy lies—you see, our body also creates antibodies to friendly foods during a process called immune tolerance.

We have a system in place that initially tags a new foreign substance (food) as questionable but, once it is deemed safe, lets our body accept it without attack. During this "evaluation" phase, IgG antibodies are also made. But here is where it gets tricky: there are four different subtypes of IgG antibodies. New evidence suggests that IgG subtype 4 (IgG4) is the antibody made to foods that we will tolerate; it will not generate an immune response. IgG subtypes 1, 2, and 3, however, will all cause an immune response. So, if we measure all subtypes of IgG, we should be able to tell if the food is being seen as a harmful invader (IgG subtypes 1–3 present) or if the food is foreign but friendly (IgG4). Significant disagreements exist between integrative medicine and traditional medicine over this concept of food testing.

I firmly believe that food sensitivity (IgG mediated) is a major culprit, not only in eczema but also in many other childhood inflammatory conditions, including asthma, ADHD, irritable bowel syndrome (IBS), and others. I also want to emphasize that when the body is in a heightened state of inflammation from poor diet, stress, environmental toxins, and the like, it will be more likely to create antibodies against safe foods. Figure 2.1 shows the most common foods we tend to form antibodies against when our immune systems are overactive.

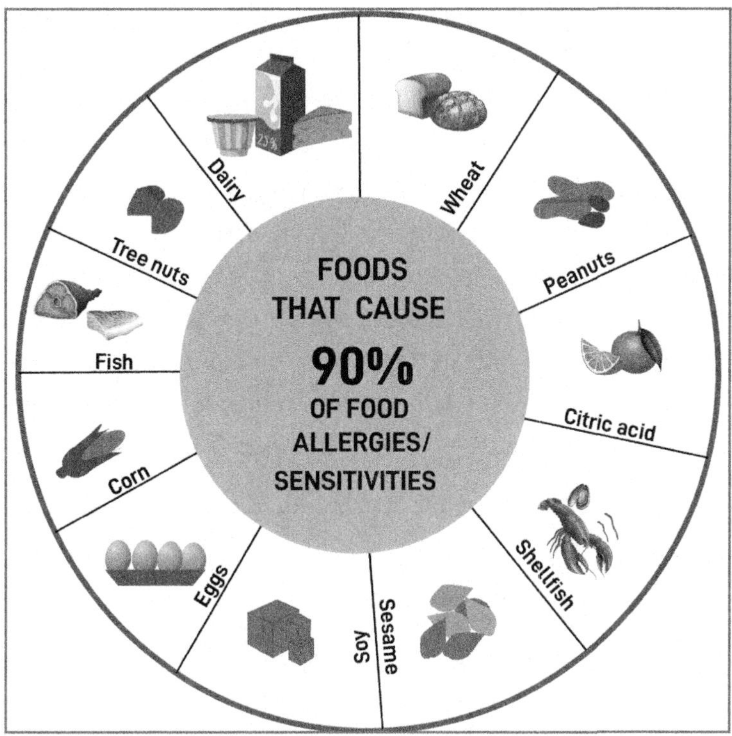

Figure 2.1

What Is *Food Intolerance*?

In food intolerance, certain individuals lack the correct enzymes to process and digest specific substances in food. The classic example is lactose, which is a sugar found in milk. Our bodies require a specific enzyme called *lactase*, which is produced in the small intestine, to break down the lactose into simpler sugars that our gut can then absorb and use for energy.

People whose small intestines do not produce lactase suffer from lactose intolerance, a condition in which undigested lactose gets passed to the large intestine. The influx of undigested lactose creates a feeding frenzy for the large bowel bacteria, which then ingest and ferment the lactose. When lactose ferments in your gut, it creates a buildup of hydrogen, methane, and carbon dioxide, leading to bloating and diarrhea. Lactose intolerance can be corrected by supplementing lactase to break down the lactose. Keep in mind though, there are many individuals who may have both a food intolerance and sensitivity to milk, meaning that simply taking a lactase supplement may correct part of the problem, but they are still creating IgG antibodies to the cow's milk. Lactose-free milk (or Lactaid supplement) is not the solution.

Of note, most adults in the world (65–70 percent) are lactose intolerant.[15] It makes me wonder if humans were really meant to drink cow's milk! (More on this in Chapter 6: Dairy.)

A Key Interaction

The interplay between the three types of food reactions discussed above is complex, still only partially understood, and truly an enigma of modern medicine. The reality is that there is likely overlap between the three issues, and that is why the terms have become intermixed and confusing. (Gluten, for example, could cause an intolerance or lead to a sensitivity called celiac disease, and it can be difficult to determine which category to place it in.)

We know there is a close interplay between true food allergies and eczema, as the presence of one is much more likely to mean the presence of the other. But we are just beginning to understand how all three truly interact to contribute to eczema.

The bottom line is that no food allergy or sensitivity test is 100 percent reliable (or even 90 percent reliable). Given this discrepancy, the most reliable way to determine an issue with food is to eliminate the problem food and see if the condition improves. Although any individual can be intolerant to a plethora

---

15 https://pubmed.ncbi.nlm.nih.gov/28690131/

of foods, it turns out that certain foods tend to be the most common culprits. So the easiest (and cheapest) way to start is to temporarily remove those foods from your child's diet. Then, progressively reintroduce the desirable foods once the gut has healed to determine which foods are problematic.

Most of my families realize that once they have given up certain problematic junk foods, they have no need to reintroduce them down the road. So it's a win-win for the gut. Also, our taste buds regenerate every 30 days, so many of the cravings for food that has been removed will simply disappear over time—patience is key.

A Word of Caution

One of the biggest mistakes families make with food elimination diets is that they progressively remove the concerning foods without replacing them with nutritionally equivalent foods. For example, if spinach is removed from a child's diet because of histamine concerns, it should be replaced with kale. If nuts are removed from the diet, they should be replaced with olives or pumpkin seeds.

> Note: The Eczema Pantry section at the end of the book provides wonderful pantry replacements to lower inflammation. Chapter 8 on histamines also provides food replacement options for high histamine foods.

There is a real danger to food eliminations done without expert guidance. Readily available over-the-counter food allergy testing kits often steer families toward excessive eliminations. Following these types of test results, children may become malnourished (which prevents eczema from healing), parents could become orthorexic (fearful of food), and picky eating emerges as a real problem. This is exactly why I created the online Eczema Transformation Program with personalized weekly guidance from a Health Coach and myself. In our online community, you will be working together with a pediatrician who is aware of the pitfalls of elimination diets, who is an expert in children's nutritional needs, and who has helped thousands of families heal their children.

Now back to my son, Jake, and the recurrent eczema on his chest and back. Because we had tried some elimination diets with him and were not certain which foods were problematic, we proceeded with food sensitivity (IgG) testing. His results are in Figure 2.2.

Jake's Food Test Results

	ALLERGY			SENSITIVITY					
DIETARY ANTIGEN	IgE	IgE (µg/mL)	IMMUNE TOLERANCE TO IgE	IgG4	IgG4 (µg/mL)	IgG	IgG (µg/mL)	C3D	C3D (µg/mL)
Almond		0.19	YES	MODERATE	1.09		0.81		0.00
Apple		0.00			0.02		0.00		0.00
Asparagus		0.00			0.00		0.00	LOW	0.52
Aspergillus Mix	LOW	0.16			0.00		4.07		0.00
Cantaloupe	MODERATE	0.80			0.02		0.00		0.00
Carrot	MODERATE	0.61			0.00		0.00		0.11
Casein	MODERATE	0.80	YES	LOW	0.92		0.00		0.00
Cashew		0.00		MODERATE	1.89		0.00		0.00
Cauliflower		0.00			0.00		0.00		0.00
Celery		0.00			0.00		0.00		0.00
Cherry		0.00			0.00		0.00		0.00
Chicken		0.00			0.00		0.00		0.00
Cinnamon		0.00			0.00	LOW	1.55	LOW	0.60
Clam	HIGH	11.34		HIGH	4.07	HIGH	34.25	HIGH	3.76
Coconut		0.00			0.00		0.00		0.00
Codfish		0.00		LOW	0.26		0.00		0.00
Coffee		0.00			0.00		0.22		0.11
Corn		0.00		LOW	0.06		0.00		0.00
Cottonseed		0.00			0.00		0.00		0.00
Cow's Milk	LOW	0.61	YES	MODERATE	2.03		15.98		0.00
Crab		0.00			0.00		0.00		0.00
Cucumber		0.00			0.00		0.00		0.00
Egg Albumin	MODERATE	14.24	YES	MODERATE	15.99	MODERATE	48.15	MODERATE	6.27
Egg Yolk	LOW	0.22	YES	LOW	1.50	LOW	0.85	HIGH	7.99
English Walnut		0.00			0.00		0.15	LOW	7.13
Tomato		0.00			0.00		0.00		0.00
Tuna	LOW	0.19			0.00		0.00		0.00
Turkey	HIGH	1.70			0.00		0.00		0.00
Vanilla	LOW	0.06			0.00		0.89		0.00
Watermelon		0.00			0.00		0.00	LOW	0.23
White Potato	LOW	0.03			0.00		0.00	LOW	2.08
Whole Wheat		0.00		MODERATE	0.16		0.00		0.03
Yellow Squash	LOW	0.16	YES	LOW	0.19		0.00		0.00

Figure 2.2

I won't go into detail about the intricacies of Jake's labs, but he was reacting to dairy, gluten, turkey, almonds, clams, and eggs. We don't eat clams often in our family, but he was eating a turkey sandwich almost every day for lunch, in addition to lots of eggs, almonds, cashews, cow's milk, and gluten. So we eliminated (replaced) these foods for several months, and his resultant skin changes were amazing.

It was definitely hard for him to remove these—as a high school kid, he was often out with friends and eating on the road. But Jake felt empowered to make his food decisions and embraced his goal of clear skin and going shirtless at the pool. He gained confidence as we watched his skin clear. After we healed his gut with my Eczema Transformation Protocol, we started adding these foods back one at a time. Some (cow's milk and gluten) we have not been able to bring back, as they cause symptoms every time. Now he is aware of the foods that cause his eczema issues to resurface and can decide for himself whether to eat those. Occasionally, he will gorge on pizza, knowing that it may cause a flare—but to him it's worth it.

Although the last dietary changes are what cleared up Jake's skin, diet was just one part of his eczema solution. One thing Jake underestimated was how much stress was contributing to his eczema. Stress in our lives causes hormonal changes that can affect our inflammatory state. It's really our overall inflammatory state that determines whether eczema manifests itself on our skin. In the next chapter, we will look at our body's level of inflammation and what I like to term *the inflammatory bucket*.

Chapter Takeaways

- The three primary terms used when discussing issues with food are food allergy, food sensitivity, and food intolerance.
- Acute food allergy is a potentially life-threatening allergic response to certain foods (e.g., peanuts and shellfish) mediated through IgE antibodies, and is diagnosed with skin testing.
- Food sensitivity, mediated through less acute IgG antibodies, plays a central role in eczema development and is diagnosed with a food elimination diet or with blood testing.
- In food intolerance, certain individuals lack the correct enzymes to process and digest specific substances in food, as in lactose intolerance.

For more information about food allergy testing or our Eczema Transformation Program, please visit the book resource page by scanning the QR code below.

3

The Inflammatory Bucket

I have practiced medicine long enough that few cases truly stump me—but that changed when I met Bella. Bella was a beautiful 15-month-old who was curious and playful, running around the room with boundless energy. She was a typical toddler with a major exception—she did not have one hair anywhere on her body. Every hair on her body had fallen out about six months earlier. Bella, of course, had no idea that she was different and was totally content without hair, but her parents were not so lucky.

Her parents, Mark and Kerry, had been able to cope with her recurrent ear infections, upper respiratory infections, eczema flares, and food allergies. But once all of Bella's hair fell out, their coping mechanisms just couldn't keep up. Kerry said to me, "People keep asking us about Bella's cancer treatments, or say they are sorry about the cancer. But she doesn't have cancer!" As her mom said this, Bella looked up and smiled at a toy she'd found in the corner, and I realized that she didn't even have eyebrows.

As I delved further into Bella's story, I realized the hair loss was just the tip of the iceberg. In her short life, Bella had already suffered five ear infections (all treated with antibiotics), an upper respiratory infection with Respiratory Syncytial Virus (RSV), eczema, and food allergies. (Of note, 80 percent of ear infections resolve without antibiotics).[16] The family's stress mounted as her issues worsened, and both Bella's mom and dad worried about the implications of all the medications she was taking. Mark and Kerry, however, didn't see the connection between childhood illnesses and skin issues. They asked, "What do her ear infections have to do with eczema and hair loss?" Mark and Kerry were not seeing the larger issue lurking beneath the surface (see Figure 3.1).

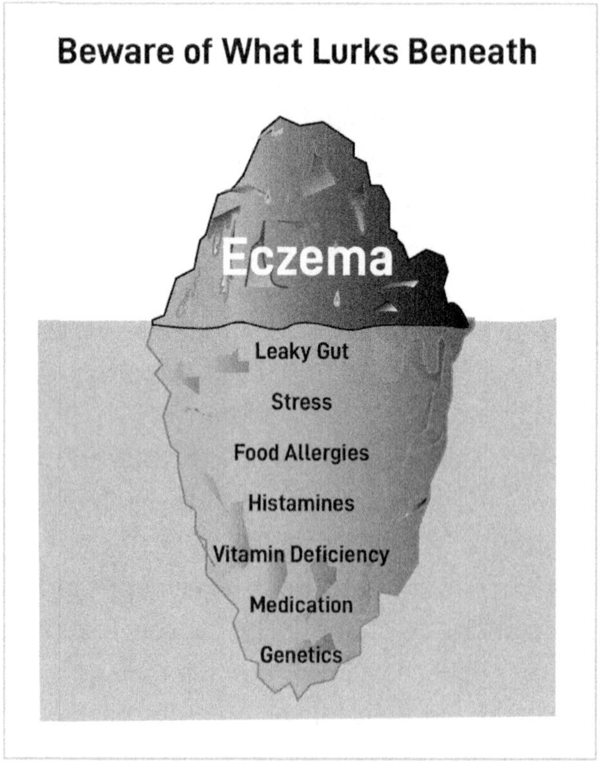

Figure 3.1

[16] https://pubmed.ncbi.nlm.nih.gov/14973951/

The much larger process I am referring to is inflammation. Although Bella appeared to have an isolated skin problem (loss of hair and eczema), she actually had a more concerning issue—runaway inflammation. You are probably wondering how a 15-month-old could have that amount of inflammation in her body. There is not just one factor leading to this inflammatory storm. We all maintain a certain amount of inflammation that our bodies will tolerate. In fact, inflammation is an important part of our normal immune system; it allows us to fight infections, heal cuts and bruises, and mend broken bones. But in patients with eczema, that inflammatory process goes haywire because of dozens of factors in our lives and environments. We refer to these types of diseases, caused by overactive immune systems, as autoimmune diseases.

The analogy I like to use with autoimmune disease is the inflammatory bucket. The bucket will "hold" a certain amount of inflammation in each person. The size of the bucket is determined by many factors, including age, genetics, sex, ethnicity, environment, and even the country we are born in. (Children born outside of the United States are 50 percent less likely to develop eczema.)[17] Each time our bodies encounter certain foods, toxins, allergens, chemicals, stress, and many other factors we will discuss in this book, it adds to the bucket.

It's more than the one thing that finally overflowed the bucket—it's the multitude of things that filled the bucket in the first place.

Once the bucket is full, the next inflammatory drop to be added will result in autoimmune disease. For example, it may seem that eczema started from

[17] Silverberg JI, Simpson EL, Durkin HG, Joks R. Prevalence of allergic disease in foreign-born American children. JAMA Pediatr. 2013;167(6):554–560.[↩]

dairy, but dairy was just the next item that caused the bucket to spill over. It's more than the one thing that finally overflowed the bucket—it's the multitude of things that filled the bucket in the first place.

Filling the Bucket

As we approach eczema from this understanding, we need to examine all the factors that fill our inflammatory bucket (see Figure 3.2). We are all a bit different in how we fill the bucket. One person may have a huge inflammatory response to nuts, while another responds to gluten, and a third responds to stress. In Bella's case, she had a huge response to a leaky gut caused by antibiotics, household stress, dairy, and vaccinations. Once all these factors were tallied, her body could not manage this level of inflammation.

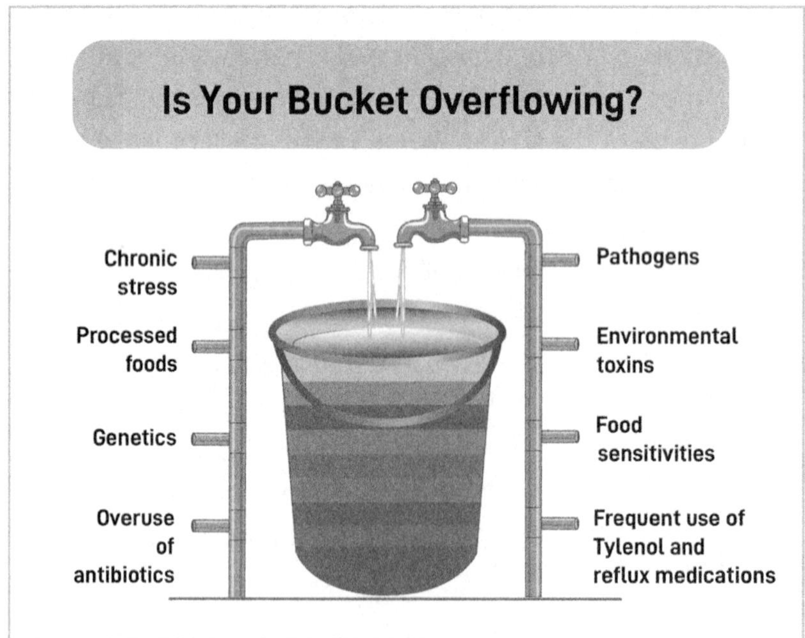

Figure 3.2

Before Mark and Kerry brought Bella to see me, they had been through the standard treatments I see from conventional medicine in America. The overall approach in our country has been to blunt the inflammatory immune response with medications without any regard for the origins of the excess inflammation. This is why Bella was given topical steroids at the first signs of eczema, and, as her eczema worsened, oral steroids. By the time she saw me, her allergist was recommending tofacitinib cream, which is a powerful immune-suppressing drug used to treat moderate to severe rheumatoid arthritis. Understandably, Mark and Kerry were scared to death to put this on their daughter's skin.

What makes this story even more interesting is that Mark and Kerry had been giving Bella Tylenol for years for fevers, and more recently, to ease her pain from eczema. Little did they know that using Tylenol (aka acetaminophen or paracetamol) drastically increases the risk of eczema, particularly in the first year of life. A 2010 study revealed that even monthly use of acetaminophen can more than double the risk, while yearly use may increase the risk by 50 percent.[18] Tylenol can cause dysfunction in the immune system (which is already problematic in these kids), although the exact mechanism is unknown. To make matters worse, it also increases the risk of asthma. The answer: don't overtreat fevers! Fevers are the body's natural way of fighting infection.

Our young couple had also used acid-suppressing medications (i.e., Zantac, Pepcid) during Bella's first year of life to treat reflux. Reflux medications like the ones above, but also including Maalox, Mylanta, Prilosec, and others, have all been shown to increase the risk of eczema and food allergies.[19] It appears that

---

18 https://www.atsjournals.org/doi/full/10.1164/rccm.201005-0757OC

19 https://www.ncbi.nlm.nih.gov/pmc/articles/PMC6137535/

the normal acidic environment in our guts is crucial for the digestion and absorption of food, and when blocked with an antacid, an inflammatory reaction occurs.

To complete Bella's perfect storm of medications related to eczema development was the use of antibiotics to treat her recurrent ear infections. Many overworked primary care doctors in our country know that it is much easier to write an antibiotic prescription for the frustrated mom with the screaming baby than to counsel her for 30 minutes on why antibiotics are most often not needed for ear infections. Those unnecessary antibiotics wreak havoc on our microbiome, knocking out all good bacteria along with the bad. Unsurprisingly, the use of antibiotics in children is associated with the development of eczema.[20]

Of note, the Centers for Disease Control and Prevention (CDC) estimate that 30 percent of all antibiotics prescribed in outpatient clinics are unnecessary.[21] And even if you aren't prescribed an antibiotic, there is a good chance you are still getting them in your diet. Of all the antibiotics sold in the United States each year, 80 percent are used in the animal industry.[22] Antibiotics used in raising animals likely play a role in the altered microbiome of every person eating that Big Mac or Whopper. So, if meat is your thing, make sure you are buying antibiotic-free products to protect those delicate little guys in your gut.

After I took Bella's medication history, I was astonished to hear that the allergist had not even asked about the use of these medications. What their allergist was missing (or ignoring) were all the factors lurking beneath the surface of little Bella's skin.

---

20 https://www.ncbi.nlm.nih.gov/pmc/articles/PMC6137535/

21 https://www.cdc.gov/antibiotic-use/stewardship-report/pdf/stewardship-report.pdf

22 https://www.fda.gov/media/94906/download

I challenge you to look deeper at what may be filling your inflammatory bucket. As you identify and modify those inflammatory factors, you are restoring your immune system to its baseline function, rather than squashing it with medication.

Bella became my patient that day and has been one of the toughest cases I have faced in my 20-year career. We have worked for two years on restoring her immune system and healing her gut through dietary changes, lifestyle adjustments, correcting vitamin and mineral deficiencies, and reducing stress. I couldn't be happier to report she recently has regrown a new, beautiful head of hair! (see Figure 3.3)

BELLA'S INFLAMMATORY BUCKET

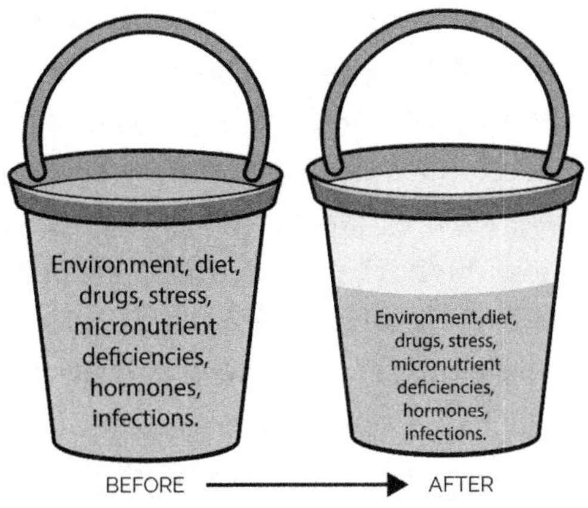

Figure 3.3

One factor I didn't mention in Bella's story is that both of her parents suffered from significant seasonal allergies for much of their lives. One might assume that Bella was destined to develop allergies herself, but maybe those genetics were just one more ingredient that was added to the bucket.

Inflammation or Genetics?

About a year ago, Bryan and Amy walked into my clinic with their lovely baby, Henry, in tow. As I pulled back the blanket of Henry's car carrier, I immediately saw why they were there—their precious baby boy was covered in eczema. I gently pulled the little guy out of the carrier and peeled off his onesie. Most of Henry's cheeks, belly, and back were covered with red patchy lesions of eczema, and he was not happy about me touching them.

Amy stated, "He is breastfeeding just fine and gaining weight, but he started breaking out in eczema a few weeks ago. And since the eczema started, sleep has gotten worse and so has bath time." I noticed Bryan nod his head, but he otherwise remained stoic with his arms crossed. After examining Henry, I asked all my usual questions about Henry's development, life at home, and their adjustment to being first-time parents.

I then began to discuss Henry's eczema and explained that 60 percent of eczema cases appear during the first year of life.[23] I also explained the inflammatory bucket and how genetic factors affect how the bucket is filled. But as I began to discuss how pregnancy and environmental factors play a role in eczema development, Bryan just started shaking his head in disbelief. Clearly, he did not like what I was saying. I asked him if something was wrong, and he replied, "Listen, my brother and I had eczema when we were kids, and so we know it's genetic. Plus, Henry is only four months old, so he hasn't been around long enough for 'environmental factors' to even play a role in this."

And with that he shrugged and mentally checked out of the appointment. I wish I could tell you this was the first time I'd heard this from a father, or even from a mother, for that matter. But dads tend to be the most absolute about it.

---

[23] https://www.ncbi.nlm.nih.gov/pmc/articles/PMC2957505/

Have you ever experienced a mild or severe illness, like thyroid issues, anxiety, or ear infections, and were told it was genetic and there was nothing you could do to prevent it? Have you ever felt helpless because you believed your genes had caused your illness? I think it's worth a discussion to determine if there was any truth in what Bryan said.

I can remember thinking most of our health issues were either genetic (defined in our DNA) or infectious (caused by some bacteria, virus, or other organism). But over the last five to ten years, I have learned that genetics may put certain individuals at risk of disease but it's their environment that causes the disease to manifest itself. Put another way: genetics loads the gun, but our environment pulls the trigger.

Much work has been done to look for the genetic origins of eczema—after all, it affects more than 20 percent of children worldwide and up to 10 percent of adults. Thus, if a genetic origin were found, it could possibly be a target for gene therapies. So let's take a look at some genetic evidence.

The most obvious evidence for a genetic link lies in the tendency for eczema to run in families.[24] Studies have indicated that the risk for a person to develop eczema can increase three to five times if one or both parents have a history of eczema.[25] Just like Bryan in the story above, it is quite common for me to see a child with eczema, and one or both parents describe a history of eczema in themselves or one of their family members. In fact, the first descriptions of eczema-type diseases in families go back 2,000 years. Ancient Romans described that Emperor Augustus (63 BC–14 AD) had dry, itchy patches on his skin and suffered

---

[24] https://pubmed.ncbi.nlm.nih.gov/15383434/

[25] https://pubmed.ncbi.nlm.nih.gov/20804468/

from a seasonal respiratory disorder, and both his grandson and his great-grandnephew suffered from similar symptoms.[26]

Beyond simply looking at families, though, we can now actually look at a human's blueprint. When the human genome was mapped in 2004, it revolutionized the genetic aspect of medicine. We can now compare the DNA of individuals with a particular disease to those without disease and look for the differences in their DNA. Also, remember that each human has two copies of a gene: one from mom and one from dad. So, even if one is damaged, the other gene may be working well.

Current Genetic Data

When this concept was applied to eczema, a mutation in the FLG gene that encodes for a protein called filaggrin showed the strongest association.[27] A mutation is a change that occurs in our DNA sequence, either because of mistakes when the DNA is copied or as the result of environmental factors. Between 20 and 30 percent of people with eczema have an FLG gene mutation. Filaggrin plays an important role in the structure of the outermost skin layer, helping to create a watertight barrier. It is also important for the skin's natural moisturizing process and for maintaining correct skin acidity (pH). When mutations in filaggrin occur, the skin barrier is defective, allowing toxins, bacteria, and substances that can cause allergic reactions (allergens), such as pollen and dust mites, to enter the skin. This is likely why patients with the FLG gene mutation are at a higher risk of contracting eczema.[28]

---

26 P.D. Mier, "Earliest description of the atopic synrome?," Br J Dermatol, (1975): 92:359.

27 https://pubmed.ncbi.nlm.nih.gov/16550169/

28 https://www.karger.com/Article/Fulltext/500402#ref13

Another gene that plays a role in the development of eczema is KIF3A, which codes for a protein involved in cell communication and transport. A mutation in this gene leads to the skin barrier becoming weakened and to water loss, both of which increase eczema risk.[29]

Third, the CARD11 gene carries the information to make a protein that is necessary for the proper functioning of white blood cells (lymphocytes). Lymphocytes are immune cells that protect the body from infections and play a role in eczema. Mutations in the CARD11 gene can result in eczema because of a weakened immune system. Researchers have identified at least five CARD11 mutations that may be present in people with eczema.[30]

Currently, more than fifty additional genes have been associated with eczema and research continues to uncover more mutations.[31] However, it's imperative to remember that association and causation are not the same thing, and so we must take these associations with a grain of salt. You will also learn below that the presence of a gene and the expression of a gene are not the same thing.

So it's possible little Henry inherited a damaged copy of one of these genes from dad, or that sometime during development, the gene mutated and developed errors. But it's also possible that the gene was not active until it was activated by some environmental factor. And this is where everything gets interesting—and murky.

You see, the information stored in our DNA is not enough to completely explain human development, physiology, and disease. The ways these genes are expressed is really what determines

---

[29] https://www.nature.com/articles/s41467-020-17895-x

[30] https://pubmed.ncbi.nlm.nih.gov/28628108/

[31] https://www.frontiersin.org/articles/10.3389/fgene.2020.00270/full

whether we develop a particular disease, and there are a lot of factors that contribute to how a gene is expressed—enter the field of epigenetics.

Epigenetics: The Answer to Nature Versus Nurture

Epigenetics is the study of how your behaviors and environment can cause changes that affect the way your genes work. Unlike genetic changes, epigenetic changes are, fortunately, reversible and do not change your DNA sequence. But they can change how your body reads a DNA sequence.

Although Henry may have inherited a damaged copy of a gene from Bryan, it may have been the antibiotics he received at birth that changed the way his genes were expressed and started the eczema process. This is likely why so many different factors have been identified as having relationships with eczema—birth factors like maternal stress and diet, C-sections, antibiotics, reflux medications, and the microbiome, to name a few.

A fascinating example of the power of epigenetics can be seen in the rodent world with Agouti mice.[32] These mice all carry something called the Agouti gene, a gene that normally encodes for a brownish or black-colored mouse—but when overactivated, produces obese mice that develop heart disease, diabetes, and cancers. Researchers took two groups of these obese, unhealthy Agouti mice that were genetically identical (had the exact same DNA) and bred them together. The only difference between the groups is what the mothers were fed while pregnant. In the control group, the mothers were fed standard mouse food, while in the experimental group the mothers ate standard mouse food

---

32 https://www.nature.com/scitable/topicpage/obesity-epigenetics-and-gene-regulation-927/

plus the supplements choline, folic acid, B12, and betaine. What the researchers found surprised them.

The mothers who had vitamin supplements added to their diet produced offspring that were thin, healthy, and had fur of a totally different color. The mothers who were fed the standard diet had the usual obese, unhealthy offspring. But when they compared the DNA of the starkly different-looking mice, it was the same in both groups. In studying the healthy offspring, the researchers found the baby mice had actually turned off the Agouti gene through a process called methylation (though the gene was still there). The vitamins had provided the molecules necessary to turn off this unhealthy portion of DNA. These results were groundbreaking because they showed that a mother can influence the expression of her child's genes simply through the diet she consumes while pregnant.

The effects have been found to be the most profound during the first trimester of pregnancy. Imagine how much of our current obesity epidemic may be related to this three-month period of pregnancy when diet has a massive influence on gene expression.

The good news here is that we have the power to alter our gene expression with our behavior and environment. Granted, you can't pick your mom and dad, but you can influence how their diseases may or may not affect you. (Unfortunately, I have not been able to influence my own father's gene expression, meaning I am habitually late and I can never find my keys.)

Our discussion so far has focused on human genetics, but we would be remiss if we didn't mention the other major genetic elephant in the room—our microbiome. You see, we each harbor nearly one thousand different species of bacteria in and on our bodies, and those bacteria contain thousands of genes that help to expand the human genome. Each of us carries a different combination of bacteria, giving us a unique microbiome fingerprint that is like no other.

And here is the crazy part: the bacterial genes affect the function and expression of our human genes. When we damage or alter our microbiome, we have downstream effects on our own gene expression.[33] Our microbiomes are inherited, just like our DNA, so it's possible that some of the "inherited" diseases we see may actually be related to our inherited microbiome as much as our inherited DNA from mom and dad. Mind blown!

As I finished up my comprehensive PowerPoint discussion on epigenetics and the human microbiome three and a half hours later, Bryan had a totally different look on his face. He was curled up in the fetal position in the corner, but at least his arms were no longer crossed. As he rose from the floor, a smile spread across his face. He said, "Doc, I guess I need to rethink my 'It's all in your genes' theory, huh?" Bryan and I both laughed, but he truly changed his mindset about the origins of eczema. The biggest beneficiary? Henry. Over the next few months, Henry's skin changed from inflamed and itchy to clear, soft baby skin. Bryan and Amy had made the necessary changes to allow Henry's skin to heal from eczema. They changed the expression of Henry's genes by altering his environment—a really powerful concept.

If you can consider for a moment that we have the power to change our genes by modifying our environment (and thereby altering the course of chronic disease), join me in the next chapter, where I travel to the other side of the world to discover the connection between our gut and our skin.

---

33 https://www.ncbi.nlm.nih.gov/pmc/articles/PMC7680557/

Chapter Takeaways

- Our bodies will tolerate a certain amount of inflammation before it begins to overflow into autoimmune disease, a concept called the inflammatory bucket.
- Common medications such as Tylenol, Zantac, and antibiotics add to the volume of our buckets and are related to eczema development.
- Although certain genetic mutations have been associated with eczema, the *expression of those genes* (epigenetics) is largely determined by our environment and is within our control.

For more help managing your inflammatory bucket, check out my book resources page by scanning the QR code below.

4

My Gut Leap of Faith

I was standing on the edge of a platform 143 feet above the icy blue water of the Kawarau River in Queenstown, New Zealand, with a bungee cord wrapped around my ankles. It was October of 2016, and we had just arrived in New Zealand after quitting our jobs, renting out our house in the U.S., and saying goodbye to all our relatives and friends.

As I shuffled my feet closer to the edge, my heart was pounding in my chest as I listened to my family cheering me on. The guide told me to look at the pre-jump camera and smile, so I obliged and attempted to look happy. After the picture, I turned back and the guide said, "Okay, JUMP!" But in those moments, I thought: *How did I wind up here? Why am I standing on the edge of a perfectly good bridge about to jump off, with only an elastic cord attached to my ankles?* The previous few weeks played like a movie in my mind.

Although my moment on the bridge occurred in Queenstown, we had moved to Wellington, New Zealand, a few weeks prior, which is much farther to the north. Within one week of our arrival, the kids were enrolled in school and John started his job with the orthopedic team at Wellington Hospital. I, on the other hand, began the waiting process for my work visa. While sitting around in my apartment overlooking the bay and the surrounding rolling green hills, I thought: *I need to reinvent myself. I finally have all this time on my hands! I should dig deeper into health topics and make educational Instagram posts because I love teaching and I am obsessed with Instagram.* I got to work.

One day while searching for info on how foods rich in vitamin D can help kids with eczema, I came across a blog post from renowned functional physician Dr. Mark Hyman entitled "Seven Strategies to Eliminate Eczema." In this article, the discussion did not revolve around topical steroids, or the latest immune-suppressing drugs. Instead, it focused on leaky gut, abnormal gut flora, and the power of the gut to treat disease. He went on to discuss how previous exposure to antibiotics increases the risk of eczema.

WHAT?? I was riveted. Based on my family's experience, I knew that food played a major role in skin conditions, but leaky gut and gut flora? Antibiotics can cause eczema? "Hold the phone!!" I exclaimed. (Yes, I talk to myself routinely.)

Because I am a complete nerd, I was overcome with joy and started learning more about this "gut" thing and its connection to all other body systems. I was blown away. "There is a specialty in medicine that focuses on nutrition and lifestyle to treat chronic disease? Incredible!" I shouted out loud to no one. I researched Dr. Hyman and learned that he was also the head of the Institute For Functional Medicine (IFM) at the Cleveland Clinic in Ohio.

Immediately, I signed up for all the IFM grand rounds and tutorials. Low and behold, I discovered a world of medicine that made perfect sense. It led me to believe that the human body can heal itself if given the proper tools. Chronic disease can be reversed if we understand the triggers that lie within our lifestyle and environment. But it would take a major leap of faith to diverge from my conventional medical training and actually start to treat patients in this new, functional way. Functional medicine determines how and why illness occurs and restores health by addressing the root causes of disease for each individual—just what I was looking for!

So, as I found myself on that bridge, looking at the water far below, I bent my knees, took a deep breath, and leaped.

Getting to the Guts of the Matter

To understand how eczema starts inside our guts, we need to understand a bit about the digestive process. This process is broken down into five basic stages:

1. Ingestion
2. Digestion
3. Absorption
4. Assimilation
5. Elimination

Stages of Digestion

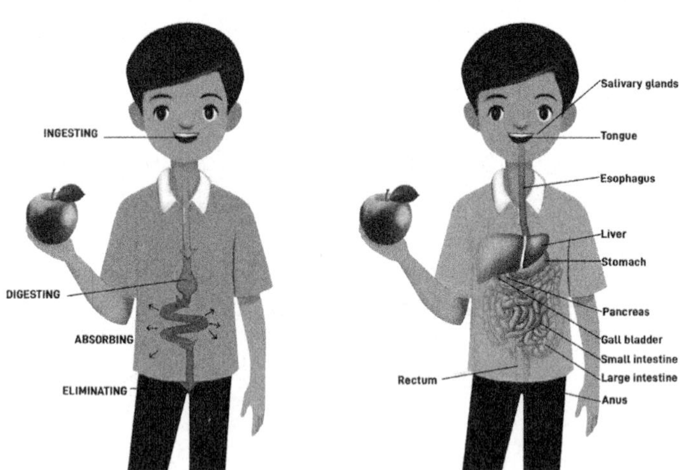

Figure 4.1

Ingestion

Ingestion starts the process and begins as we place food into our mouths. As we begin to chew, our salivary glands produce saliva to help soften our food. Our taste buds are activated to appreciate flavors and the palatability of the food. This is where the American diet first starts to wreak havoc on us. The food industry has introduced chemicals into our food that put our taste buds into a state of bliss that nature has a tough time competing with. Food scientists have figured out how to create these chemical compounds that our taste buds simply can't resist. There's a reason those first few bites of McDonald's or Doritos taste so darn wonderful.

Digestion

As the food passes down the esophagus and into the stomach and intestines, the digestion process begins. As the food is turned and churned in our bellies, the larger molecules are broken down into smaller molecules. Our cells understand a simple language I like to call the *whole foods language*. This language includes familiar words like potassium, calcium, magnesium, and other nutrients found in fruits, vegetables, meats, eggs, etc. However, when the body encounters strange new chemicals that have been added in a lab, our cells get confused. They struggle to decipher food additives like monosodium glutamate (MSG) or disodium 5'-inosinate (E631). In addition, our bodies consider some of these substances to be foreign invaders and start an inflammatory reaction to fight them. Gluten and dairy are two common culprits that push the body into defense mode.

I want to take a minute here to point out that it is ridiculous to place something called a nutrition label on many of the foods we eat. We are implying that there is nutritional value in foods that are simply garbage. Many of us are taught in school how to read parts of food labels such as fiber, fat, or sugar content, but few of us are educated on the actual ingredient list. We are bombarding our digestive system with loads of crap that the food industry has convinced us is "a nutritious part of our daily breakfast!"

The food we eat provides the fuel for our body to make the cells that sustain us. New skin cells are produced every thirty days, lung cells every eight days, and gastrointestinal cells every two days, approximately. To build these cells, our bodies require the vital nutrients that are found in fruits and vegetables. But when we give our children breakfast cereal, for example, we are supplying their cells with things like rice flour, canola oil, maltodextrin, trisodium phosphate (TSP), caramel color, and tertiary butylhydroquinone (TBHQ). Some of these chemicals are actually known to damage the gut and lead to inflammatory reactions and food allergies. More on this in Chapter 5.

Absorption

This brings us to the next step in the human nutrition cycle: absorption. As this slimy mass of squishy food particles enters our small intestine, the body is carefully evaluating and trying to break down each substance into something small and safe enough to enter our bloodstream. A whole team of specialized cells line up like soldiers along our intestines to guard this process. These guards are known as enterocytes. In a healthy gut, they look like the cells on the left in Figure 4.2, with lots of "hairs" and tight junctions with their neighbor. However, if they have been bombarded by enemy chemicals and molecules, they start to look like the pitiful guys on the right and can't hold on to the soldier next to them. These gaps that form between soldiers allow the enemy (inflammatory particles) to enter allied territory. As this process progresses, the entire gut can become "leaky" as more holes are breached through fallen soldier cells.

Our Intestinal Lining

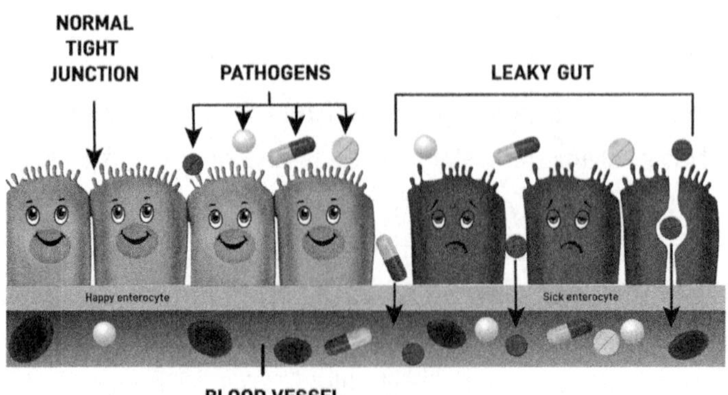

Figure 4.2

In addition to standing guard, the soldier cells also produce enzymes to aid digestion and absorption. When the cells become sick and leaky, they cannot produce enough enzymes to allow for nutrients to be absorbed and delivered to the proper cells.

This is why many parents out there get frustrated after trying various diets and food eliminations without much success. Simply modifying the diet without a focus on healing the gut will typically fail. I created my Eczema Transformation Protocol to address these issues.

Assimilation

Now that the nutrients (and other stuff) have moved into the bloodstream, our body can access them for maintenance and building. We call this assimilation. All the zinc inside that chick-pea or nut is circulating through the blood and is taken up by skin cells to keep our skin happy and healthy. Without adequate amounts of circulating nutrients, our cells wither and die. But they also suffer when the fuel is of poor quality. In kids with poor digestion and absorption, the food moves through and gets pooped out without delivering the necessary minerals and vitamins. Does your child have persistently loose poops? Do you often see lots of undigested food particles in their stool? Those can be signals that the gut is not working properly. More info on micronutrients in Chapter 9.

Elimination

The last step in our nutrition cycle is elimination—aka pooping. Pooping every day is how our body detoxifies itself from unwanted chemicals or breakdown products. When we poop too infrequently, we have a buildup of toxins. When we poop too much, we are likely eliminating valuable nutrients that haven't had time to be absorbed. Poop quality is just as important as poop quantity.

The lovely folks over in Bristol, England, took the time to create a beautiful chart on poop, called the Bristol Stool Chart (see Figure 4.3). You can compare your poops (or those of someone you love) to the seven different types to determine your poop quality. The goal is to poop AT LEAST once daily—a long soft snake (Type 4, per the chart) that comes out easily without much effort. It is normal for people to poop after each meal so long as it is Type 4.

Lastly, I cannot tell you how many kids I see who seem to be pooping fine but are, in fact, full of poop. If your child is pooping every day, but the poops are hard pebbles (Type 1), there is a problem.

BRISTOL STOOL CHART		
Type 1	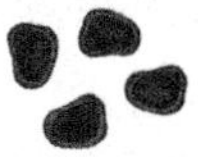	Separate hard lumps, like nuts (hard to pass)
Type 2	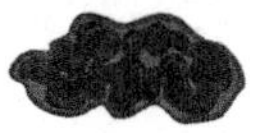	Sausage-shaped but lumpy
Type 3	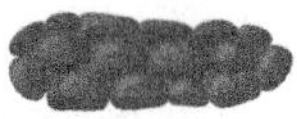	Like a sausage but with cracks on its surface
Type 4	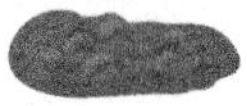	Like a sausage or snake, smooth and soft
Type 5	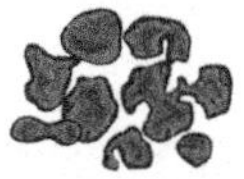	Soft blobs with clear-cut edges (passed easily)
Type 6	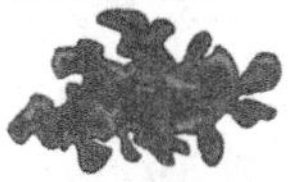	Fluffy pieces with ragged edges, a mushy stool
Type 7	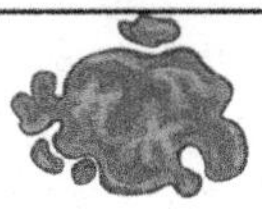	Watery, no solid pieces Entirely liquid

Figure 4.3

The Leaky Gut

Now that you are well-versed on the biology of eating and pooping, I want to focus on one of the concepts mentioned in the absorption section. Leaky gut (aka increased intestinal permeability) is the result of damage to our gut lining, which allows spaces to develop between the cells. Leaking through these spaces creates a low-grade inflammation in reaction to food particles (deemed foreign by your immune system) that literally leak through our gut wall.

The leakage of things like gluten and dairy causes food sensitivities, which in turn are some of the most common causes of eczema. Other chemicals found in highly processed foods also "leak" through our defenses, increasing the activity of our immune system.

Two-thirds of Our Immune System Resides in Our Gut

Keep in mind that two-thirds of our immune system resides in our guts, so if our gut is out of whack, so is our immune system. Because our skin is also one of the other primary immune components, the two are intimately connected—unhappy gut equals unhappy skin.

As we discussed in the food allergy chapter, we have white blood cells that float around in our blood, feeling everything they pass. When they feel something foreign that they perceive as dangerous, like a virus or a foreign food particle, they begin a cascade of events to protect the body from this invader. One of those events is to remember the shape of the invader they just encountered, and then manufacture antibodies against this shape for future defense. That's why you must first be exposed to a virus or food that your body begins to make antibodies against, so that in subsequent exposures your body is ready to react. (Again, this is why no rash occurs when you touch poison ivy for the first time in your life—but the next time, watch out! It's also why you can eat eggs for many months and years and then develop an issue.)

When the gut is leaky, many food and chemical particles that normally would not be absorbed are able to pass into the bloodstream. This presents our immune system with an overload of foreign substances to evaluate and assign a threat level to.

As more and more particles leak through, the system becomes overwhelmed and sends messages to the other immune organs (e.g., skin, bone marrow, thymus, and spleen) that the body is under attack. The skin is the body's largest elimination organ, so it's not surprising that it becomes active when toxins careen through the bloodstream. A rash or eczema is a sign that the body is trying to get rid of these toxins.

Additionally, due to the hyperactive immune process, antibodies are formed against many food molecules that are actually friendly (like nuts or soy). Sometimes, those friendly molecules are part of the body itself (this is the concept behind autoimmune diseases, like eczema and asthma). The higher the general inflammatory state, the more likely it is to create antibodies against friendly things. This is why some people tend to have multiple allergies.

So, even though it seems like some topical detergent or clothing has caused eczema, it's really the result of an immune system that is hyperactive. The red, itchy, burning skin is simply a result of the immune system performing like it should against the attack. However, we, as Americans, have become ignorant to the fact that the attacking army lies within our food. Yes, processed food and excess sugar are the proverbial Trojan horse.

Of note, our gut cells enjoy an acidic environment to work in, which is one of the reasons the use of antacid reflux medications increases the risk of eczema. The normal acidity in our gut helps the body break down food. When we disrupt the normal acidic environment, our cells struggle to break down food, further exacerbating the problem.

Other Leaky Gut Problems

Leaky gut also triggers many other problems, including fatigue, brain fog, headaches, depression, allergies, sinus problems, IBS, reflux, joint pain, skin diseases (e.g., acne and eczema), autoimmune diseases, and more. Inflammation also causes weight gain, which is triggered by insulin resistance, food sensitivities, and food allergies.

You may be reading this book for your child's eczema, but are *you* experiencing the above symptoms? Mom and Dad, you may also have a leaky gut, even though you don't have eczema as your primary issue. Most people don't associate the above symptoms like depression or headaches with their gut health, and definitely don't see any connection between their gut and immunity. Food for thought.

The Human Microbiome

In addition to housing important immune cells, our guts also host some very important guests: bacteria. Did you know that for every one human cell we have ten bacteria cells in and on our bodies? Were you aware that 3–4 pounds of an adult's weight is just bacteria?[34]

We refer to the intestinal soup of bacteria in each person's gut as their microbiome. Each individual's gut microbiome is unique, like a fingerprint or a retina, and family members tend to share very similar microbiomes. Traditionally, it has been thought that babies simply adopt their parent's microbiome, as these bacteria are passed to the growing fetus. The reality is that each baby will progressively develop their microbiome over the first few years of their life, and hundreds of different factors affect the diversity.

---

34 https://www.nih.gov/news-events/news-releases/nih-human-microbiome-project-defines-normal-bacterial-makeup-body

Evidence is mounting that the overall composition of any individual's microbiome is a significant predictor of disease risk and health issues. Correcting a *sick microbiome* (dysbiosis) is the goal of most holistic treatment regimens.

There is a continuous interplay between beneficial and potentially harmful bacteria inside our digestive system. When the balance of power shifts to the more harmful bacteria, a sick microbiome results and autoimmune diseases such as eczema, asthma, diabetes, and psoriasis develop. Taking unnecessary antibiotics for ear infections or a cough can devastate the balance of power between those bacterial groups and lead to the emergence of an autoimmune disease. In addition to antibiotics, other medications, food, stress, and environmental toxins can all shift the balance of power (see Figure 4.4).

Factors Causing Gut Bacterial Imbalance

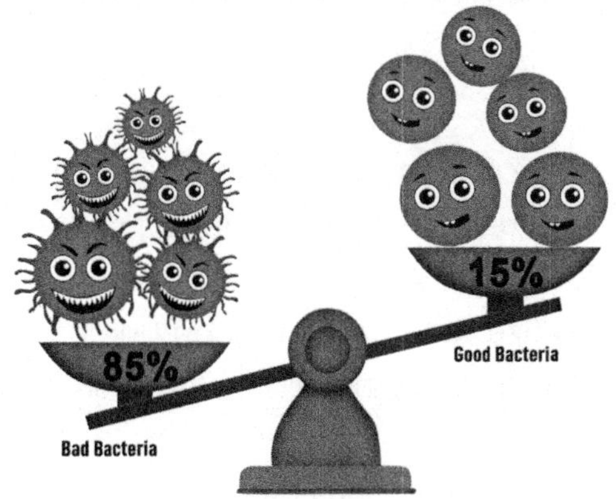

Antibiotics
Medications
Food
Stress
Environmental Toxins

Figure 4.4

In my Eczema Transformation Program, we heal the gut and allow good bacteria to repopulate our digestive system, shifting the balance back to good bacteria and clearer skin (Figure 4.5).

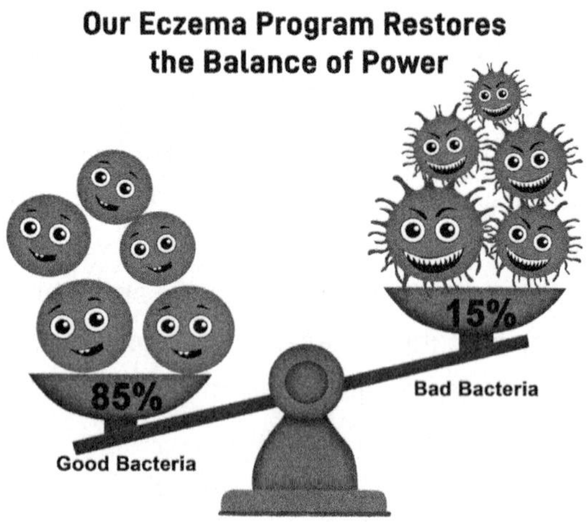

Figure 4.5

The human microbiome begins to develop the moment you are born. One bacterium in particular—*Bifidobacterium longum Subspecies infantis* (aka *B. infantis*)—is usually one of the first bacteria to colonize the infant gut, and one of the most vital. Infants normally get these bacteria from their mothers during the birth process.

Okay, now it's time to discuss some of the not-so-glamorous aspects of childbirth. When giving birth, many mothers will have an inadvertent bowel movement—and babies are typically born face down. *B. infantis* loves to live in airtight spaces like mom's colon. Hopefully, you are getting the picture. It appears babies are meant to get some of mom's poop in their mouths. Yucky stuff, right? Nature is not concerned with yucky, but nowadays many moms will prep for delivery with an enema or bowel prep to decrease the possibility of a childbirth BM. But you actually might be hurting your baby by not allowing them the full poop immersion experience!! The other major factor keeping babies from enjoying this experience is the overuse of C-section births.

C-section mania

The United States has one of the highest C-section rates in the world. We also have the honor of offering the most expensive C-section rates.[35] (The U.S. has the highest average cost for a C-section in the world.) Most people don't associate C-section with the development of childhood diseases like eczema, but the link has been established.[36]

According to figures from the CDC's latest figures, 31.9 percent of all U.S. childbirths in 2019 were delivered via C-section.[37] In 1991, C-sections only made up about 23.5 percent of births in the U.S. Working with 2009 data from 593 hospitals nationwide, a review found that cesarean rates varied tenfold across hospitals, from 7.1 percent to 69.9 percent. Even for women with low-risk pregnancies, cesarean rates varied fifteenfold, from 2.4 percent to 36.5 percent.[38] The U.S. is not alone in its high percentage of C-section deliveries—from 1990 to 2014, there was a 12.4 percent increase in the global average C-section delivery rate, according to a 2016 study.[39]

We are a society of convenience, and thus scheduling our elective C-section is easier than waiting for a heel-dragging baby to make his or her way out. But we also face a highly litigious environment in which obstetricians are much more likely to rush

---

35 https://doi.org/10.1016/S0140-6736(18)31928-7
36 https://doi.org/10.1016/j.jaci.2020.09.042
37 https://www.cdc.gov/nchs/fastats/delivery.htm
38 https://pubmed.ncbi.nlm.nih.gov/23459732/
39 https://www.ncbi.nlm.nih.gov/pmc/articles/PMC4743929/

to cesarean under the premise that waiting and having a potentially poor outcome will increase the likelihood of a lawsuit. It's a medical catch-22 for them, although this doesn't explain how rates of C-section among hospitals can vary from 7 percent to over 70 percent. We can educate mothers, families, and physicians on the clear health benefits of a vaginal delivery whenever possible and reward hospitals for maintaining appropriate ratios of vaginal to cesarean deliveries.

Adding fuel to the fire is the fact that mothers are given antibiotics at the time of C-section to reduce the high risk of infections from this procedure. As mentioned above, this can have dramatic effects on the development of the fledgling microbiome. This is one of the many reasons why *B. infantis* bacteria is disappearing from the guts of babies born in industrialized nations. It's more than a coincidence that, as the presence of *B. infantis* has gone down, the rates of autoimmune diseases in kids have gone up dramatically.

Last, *B. infantis* is an incredibly picky eater. Human breast milk is filled with something called HMOs—not a bunch of administrators in suits but rather human milk oligosaccharides. This is a carbohydrate in breast milk that appears to have the sole function of feeding the *B. infantis* bacteria. Humans can't digest it. Let me say that again—this bacteria is so important that human breast milk has evolved over time to carry food that only feeds this super bacteria in our gut! The perfect symbiotic relationship.

As bacteria eat the HMOs, a super-specialized cascade of events occurs. The bacterial genes break down the HMOs into a number of valuable growth, development, anti-inflammatory, and anti-pathogen products. HMOs themselves have been shown to be important players in the infant development game, lowering the incidence of a severe neonatal intestinal disease called necrotizing enterocolitis (NEC)—which, once again, reinforces the importance of breastfeeding.

An abnormal gut microbiome during infancy has been linked to increased risk of developing acute and long-term inflammatory diseases, such as colic, asthma and allergies, eczema, type 1 diabetes, obesity, and celiac disease.[40, 41, 42] This is supported by studies that provide strong evidence that alterations in gut microbiome composition contribute to abnormal development of the immune system and can lead to greater risk of the onset and progression of various autoimmune and allergic diseases. Therefore, understanding and protecting the gut microbiome in babies could possibly help us prevent future disease in adults.

The Gut-Healing Process

Much of what I discuss in this book relates to my overall approach to healing the gut, which in turn allows the skin to heal. Hopefully I have convinced you that providing a hospitable environment is key for maintaining a healthy gut microbiome. That's why in my eczema program we start with gut healing by first correcting diet, stress, and micronutrient deficiencies.

As the gut is beginning to heal, I then add specific digestive enzymes to support the sick intestinal cells and resolve leaky gut. Finally, once we have healed the gut and created the ideal bacterial environment, we start probiotics. Again, starting probiotics before addressing the diet is a waste of time and money.

Remember, you can't supplement your way out of a bad diet!

When choosing a probiotic, there are a number of considerations. First and foremost, only buy probiotics that are third-party

[40] https://academic.oup.com/femsle/article/366/9/fnz020/5376496?login=true
[41] https://pubmed.ncbi.nlm.nih.gov/25413686/
[42] https://onlinelibrary.wiley.com/doi/abs/10.1002/dmrr.2790

tested! (See more in Chapter 9 about choosing supplements and third-party testing.) The price point of probiotics is high compared to other supplements, so you want to be confident that the pill actually contains what the manufacturer claims.

To simplify things, we can divide probiotics into lactic acid-producing bacterial strains or spore-producing bacterial strains.

Lactic Acid Probiotics

These are probably the best-known of the probiotics and include bacteria such as *lactobacillus* and *bifidobacterium*. Through the fermentation process, they all produce lactic acid by eating lactose, sugar, and carbohydrates. The acid produced lowers gut pH (makes it more acidic) and therefore limits the growth of pathogens and *candida* (yeast).

These bacteria are transient; they do their work while they pass through the gut, rather than setting up shop for the long term. They are also sensitive to light and heat and to the acid in your stomach, so how they are manufactured and stored is important—another reason to use third-party-tested supplements.

Spore Probiotics

The bacteria in spore probiotics are able to form protective capsules, called spores, which protect the bacteria under harsh conditions. Much like the seed of a plant, the spore waits for the perfect conditions before beginning to sprout. These are colonizing bacteria that set up long-term residency in the gut. They can also go dormant until optimal nutrients are available.

One concern with spores is that they can be opportunistic and cause issues in certain environments. If your child is immunocompromised, or has a seriously weakened microbiome, these guys could take over as they colonize and cause a bigger issue.

The bacterial strains that are spore-forming typically start with *bacillus*, such as *bacillus coagulans*, *bacillus subtilis*, and *bacillus clausii*. Current studies do not suggest one is better than the other. My Eczema Transformation Program uses a lactic acid probiotic that contains two strains that have been studied extensively in kids and pregnant mothers. There are as many studies showing a beneficial reduction in eczema as there are that show no change at all. The problem with many of the studies is that the only intervention is starting probiotics. In other words, taking probiotics without changing the diet has not been shown to make much difference in a lot of studies.

As I explained above, introducing probiotics to a sick and leaky gut is likely to be a losing proposition. That's why healing the gut first is so important. Once the gut is healed, I firmly believe probiotics are beneficial to rebalance the microbiome. Entire books have been written on probiotics and the detailed benefits of each bacterial strain. However, for the purposes of transforming eczema, probiotics are just one piece of the larger puzzle. Probiotics alone will not resolve eczema.

Listening to My Gut

As I sit here, writing and reminiscing about that day on the bridge in 2016, I take solace in the fact that I have treated thousands of patients with my "gut health" leap of faith. I have discovered that more and more of the diseases that plague American children actually start in the gut—though often their symptoms do not. As a traditional doctor, I was trained to work one-on-one with patients and families. Because I could not keep up with all the requests, I took yet another leap into the unknown and created an online Eczema Transformation Program with an online community of like-minded parents. It was scary, and the learning curve was steep. But after hundreds of children and their families healed their skin with my proven method, I realized that my leap was necessary. For eczema, my motto has become: *Don't just treat the skin, heal the gut within.* Join me in the next chapter to tackle the number one culprit of the leaky gut epidemic.

Chapter Takeaways

- When we eat, an elaborate digestive process breaks down the food, evaluates all the food molecules, and absorbs nutrients through cells that line our gut.
- Damage to the cells lining the gut caused by poor dietary choices, medications, and other environmental factors leads to a leaky gut, causing our bodies to mount an inflammatory reaction to our food.
- The bacteria that reside in our gut—termed the microbiome—play a critical role in our gut health, immune system, and many other important processes in our body. Damage to the microbiome has been linked to eczema.

For more information on my signature gut healing process in The Eczema Transformation Program, scan the QR code below.

5

The Not-So-Sweet Story of Sugar

You have probably heard the old adage about the farmer who couldn't grow his own grass, or the cobbler whose children had no shoes. How about the pediatrician with chronically sick kids? That was me at the beginning of my eczema journey with my children.

John and I both had lifelong dreams of visiting Italy and wandering the streets of Rome. We finally had the opportunity to take our big trip (John actually took more than five days off work for the first time), and we left the kids with my mom and aunt. Our lives at that point consisted of 80-hour workweeks, three young children, and generalized chaos. Meals were whatever we could heat up in ten minutes. Our pantry and fridge were stocked with ready-made meals like mac and cheese, cereal, frozen burritos, frozen pizzas, and crackers—lots of crackers.

John and I rushed in the door after ten days away from our babies, and I rushed to hug my 5-year-old daughter. As I squeezed her in my arms, she cried out in pain. I looked down, and her arms and legs were covered in red, scaly bumps that were bleeding and had pus oozing out of them. I was shocked. I removed her shirt, to find half her belly covered in the same red, crusting lesions. I asked what had happened, and she just said, "Mommy, my arms hurt." I was crushed. Before I left for the trip, she just had very mild eczema to which we religiously applied topical steroids daily. How did this get so bad so quickly?

We ran to see one of my colleagues at the Saturday pediatric clinic my practice offered. My partner put my daughter on antibiotics for the infections and an oral steroid for the eczema, but I left the office terribly unsettled. Although the treatment she was given was considered "standard of care" (it still is, by the way), something wasn't right. My colleague never asked about diet, predisposing factors, home environment, or stress.

Have you ever left your doctor's office and just felt unsettled about the visit? You wondered if your doctor really heard what you were saying? I believe mothers have an incredibly strong intuition that is pretty reliable, and they know when things are amiss with their child. So began my years-long journey to uncover the source of my children's eczema and sickness.

My revelation? Sugar and processed foods were the most significant factors leading to my family's sickness. Let me tell you why.

In his pivotal book *Sugarproof*, Dr. Michael Goran details why kids love sugar so much.[43] "Their inborn love of sweet tastes makes evolutionary sense. It ensures that infants will like breast milk, which is sweet. As they start to wean, their preference for sweets helps them avoid bitter-tasting foods that could harm them."

But this innate affinity for sugar has consequences in a society that packs added sugar into so many foods. Goran also notes, "a staggering 70 percent of all packaged foods at the grocery store contain some kind of added sugar—for snack foods the number rises to 80 percent." And the tricky part is that many

---

[43] https://sugarproofkids.com/

of the foods with lots of added sugar aren't necessarily "sweet" foods. Rather, food companies add sugar or sweeteners to mask the taste of other chemicals and preservatives. Canned soups, bread, and salad dressings are great examples.

My husband ran into this problem when he was trying to change his diet and improve his health. He started eating protein bars for his snack rather than junk food, thinking that the protein content would better satiate his appetite. This was long before the FDA required the "added sugar" line on the nutrition label, and John was much more focused on the protein content of the bar than on the sugar. Turns out, he was eating "healthy" protein bars with nearly 10 grams of added sugar—as much as many energy drinks!

I discovered a number of games the food industry has been playing with us over the years. Remember the 1980s and '90s, when we were told that fats were the real problem, and as long as we ate a low-fat diet, our health would benefit? It turns out when you remove all the fat from foods, they don't taste very good. So how do you make that low-fat food palatable? Pack it with sugar and get the medical community to support the change with convincing studies.

The problem is, a number of studies that supposedly "proved" that sugar was okay and fat was the problem were sponsored by sugar companies producing high-fructose corn syrup. These studies have subsequently been disproven, but to make matters worse, we have seen a calculated series of steps by the sugar industry to cloud the matter. The sugar companies knew that the more they could blame fat, the more their product would get packed into food. The result has been not only the obesity epidemic but also chronic illness in our children and epidemic proportions of eczema.

Most of us don't see an immediate connection between sugar intake and our skin, but the evidence is clear; the daily amount of sugar you ingest directly affects your skin. And guess which nation ingests more sugar than nearly every other country, and carries the world's highest childhood obesity rates? Yes, the United States of Sugar. It's worth looking into our country's sugar epidemic so you can appreciate how large the problem is and why your child is likely affected.

Sugar Nation

During the early years of American life, the average amount of sugar consumed in the 1700s was just 4 lbs per year, which is about 1 teaspoon per day. By 2000, American sugar consumption topped out at nearly 150 lbs of sugar per person each year, which is about 45 teaspoons per day![44] The current recommendation from the American Heart Association is less than 6 teaspoons per day for children over 2, and no added sugar for children under 2 years old.[45]

To give you some perspective, a 12-ounce can of Coca-Cola contains about 9 teaspoons of sugar, and a 12-ounce Mountain Dew contains 11 teaspoons. Can you imagine putting 11 teaspoons of sugar into your morning coffee? That bowl of Kellogg's Honey Smacks gives you a nice smack in the face with 4 teaspoons per cup (and most cereal bowls hold more than a cup). So, it may not be news to you that we are overloading our children with sugar, but you may not know what sugar does to your skin.

---

[44] https://www.ers.usda.gov/webdocs/outlooks/39247/11624_sss249_4_.pdf?v=1103

[45] https://www.hsph.harvard.edu/nutritionsource/2016/08/23/aha-added-sugar-limits-children/

Sugar affects your skin in at least three significant ways:

1. High sugar intake causes insulin to spike. Insulin is the hormone our bodies produce to aid the uptake of sugar into cells. Over time, the large insulin spikes seen after ingestion of added sugars causes the increased production of several inflammatory molecules in the body. These inflammatory molecules then roam through the body, causing issues in the airways (asthma), skin (eczema), and gut.
2. High sugar intake knocks your gut out of whack by encouraging the growth of sugar-loving yeast. Overgrowth of yeast upsets the delicate balance of the microbiome in your gut, as discussed in Chapter 4. This can lead to leaky gut syndrome, which allows harmful substances into the bloodstream and the corresponding inflammatory reaction from your body. Additionally, some yeast can limit the absorption of healthy nutrients the body needs, further exacerbating the problem.
3. High sugar intake causes direct damage to skin. Chronically high levels of sugar (glucose) in the bloodstream cause excess sugar molecules to start binding to other proteins in our skin. This binding process, called glycation, damages the protein to which it attaches. Two of the commonly affected proteins in our skin are called collagen and elastin (you may have heard of celebrities getting collagen injected in their faces). Damaged collagen and elastin molecules can no longer function to support the skin, which then becomes dry and cracked, as seen in eczema. These damaged proteins are referred to as advanced glycation end products (AGEs), as seen in Figure 5.1.

Long-Term Effect of Sugar on Skin

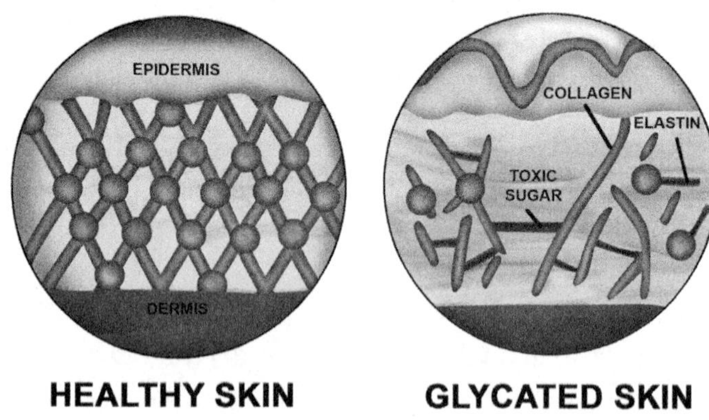

Figure 5.1

AGEs have, in many ways, become the new villains in the context of skin and aging. Interestingly, the process of glycation is also what causes bread and other high-carb foods to turn brown when you toast them. For the purposes of eczema, AGEs are simply adding one more log to the fire of inflammatory processes occurring in affected children's skin.

Even in my own children, I have watched a weekend of bingeing and poor diet choices turn into eczema outbreaks, and more acne-type reactions as they have gotten older. The immediacy of the effect is uncanny. My teenage son is now so self-conscious of the effects of sugar on his skin that he routinely turns down offers of sweets and sodas from his friends. (Score one for Mom!) And moms, before you go blaming your husbands for purchasing all the sugary foods, listen to this fact: maternal intake of added sugar during pregnancy increases the risk of childhood eczema. Unfortunately, routinely giving in to those sugar cravings during pregnancy may have played a role in your child's eczema development. (It's okay, I didn't know either.)

To help battle the problem, in 2020 the FDA began implementing new food and beverage labels (see Figure 5.2) to state how much added sugar each food product contains.

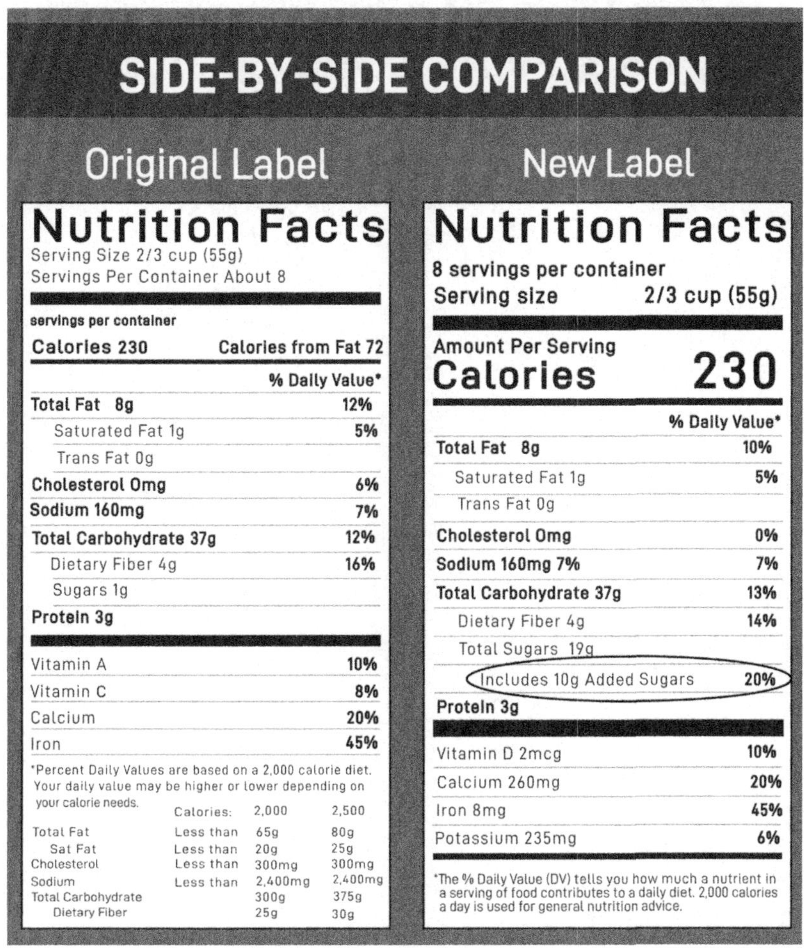

Figure 5.2

But don't forget, sugar lurks everywhere in our food and has many different names. Following is a list of 76 alternate names for sugar found in "healthy" and "organic" foods that can fool you (see Figure 5.3). Of note, there currently are more than 260 names for sugar.

76 DIFFERENT NAMES FOR SUGAR		
Agave nectar	Dextrin	Maltol
Allulose	Dextrose	Maltose
Anhydrous dextrose	Diastatic malt	Mannose
Barbados sugar	Diatase	Maple syrup
Barley malt	Ethyl maltol	Molasses
Barley malt syrup	Evaporated cane juice	Muscovado
Beet sugar	Free-flowing brown sugars	Nectar
Brown sugar	Fructose	Palm sugar
Buttered syrup	Fruit juice	Pancake syrup
Cane juice	Fruit juice concentrate	Panela
Cane juice crystals	Galactose	Panocha
Cane sugar	Glucose	Powdered sugar
Caramel	Glucose syrup solids	Raw sugar
Carob syrup	Golden sugar	Refiner's syrup
Castor sugar	Golden syrup	Rice syrup
Coconut palm sugar	Grape sugar	Saccharose
Coconut sugar	High-fructose corn syrup	Sorghum syrup
Confectioner's sugar	Honey	Sucrose
Corn sweetener	Icing sugar	Sweet sorghum
Corn syrup	Isoglucose	Syrup
Corn syrup solids	Invert sugar	Table sugar
Crystalline fructose	Lactose	Treacle
D-ribose	Malt	Turbinado sugar
Date sugar	Malt syrup	White granulated sugar
Dehydrated cane juice	Maltodextrin	Yellow sugar
Demerara sugar		

Figure 5.3

Alternatives to Sugar Explained

To reduce our sugar consumption, a number of sugar alternatives have emerged—although many are problematic for other reasons. In general, sugar directly from whole fruits also contains fiber, vitamins, minerals, and antioxidants. It really is the best form of sugar intake. My recommendation is to ensure that the only added sugar in a child's diet comes from whole fruits. Given that about 6–10 percent of all U.S. households are in a "food desert" (areas with limited or no access to healthy foods), this can be challenging for many families.[46] Thus, I think it's important to have a basic understanding of sugar and its alternatives.

Let's first address the 500-lb gorilla in the United States—high-fructose corn syrup (HFCS). The federal government was complicit in getting us addicted to this gem, as it gave huge subsidies to farmers to grow corn and levied taxes on imported pure cane sugar. HFCS quickly became the cheap alternative that food companies used to sweeten their products. Coke and Pepsi both changed from sugar to HFCS in the early 1980s because it was so much cheaper. (Fun fact: Europe does not allow colas to be sweetened with HFCS because of its detrimental health effects.)

Our bodies deal with sugar (sucrose) and fructose in very different ways. The liver is the only organ that can break down fructose, and when it encounters HFCS, it gets overwhelmed. It begins to rapidly turn the fructose into fat, leading to fatty liver disease and all the downstream health effects, including ones that impact the skin. I consider natural sugars with high levels of fructose in the same way as HFCS. These include fruit juice concentrates, fruit sugars (concentrates evaporated to crystalline form), and agave syrup. For example, many children's gummy supplements are "made with real fruit," but the fruit sugars may still be detrimental.

Even though whole fruit contains fructose, it does not put the same pressure on the liver. Fruits are loaded with fiber and water and have significant chewing resistance. For this reason, most fruits (like apples) take a while to eat and digest, meaning that the fructose hits the liver slowly. Plus, fruit is incredibly filling

[46] https://www.ers.usda.gov/webdocs/publications/82101/eib-165.pdf?v=3395.3

and contains vitamins and minerals. Eating an apple, with its 13 grams of fructose, is more filling and nutritious than a Coke, which contains 30 grams of fructose.[47, 48] Our obesity problem is compounded by the fact that the Coke drinker is still hungry after finishing.

As more data emerge about the negative health effects of excess sucrose and fructose, the food company chemists have been hard at work formulating alternate sweeteners to please our palates. Many of these sweeteners have been around for ages but are getting resurrected and refined as potentially healthier options. However, proceed with caution because *these are still considered added sugar*! Let's take a look at some common sweeteners.

Natural Sugars with Lower Fructose

- **Date sugar and date syrup:** These come from date palm trees and contain fiber, potassium, copper, iron, manganese, magnesium, and vitamin B6. By retaining some of the benefits of the whole fruit, particularly fiber, date products may slow the rise in blood sugar after ingestion.
- **Raw, dark, local honey:** Made by bees from plant nectar, honey may have been the first sweetener used by humans. It is full of enzymes, antioxidants, iron, zinc, potassium, calcium, phosphorus, vitamin B6, riboflavin, and niacin. Typically, the darker the honey, the more nutrient-dense it is. Local honey provides you with oral tolerance to local pollen, meaning it can help reduce reactions to pollen and help with seasonal allergies. Of note, honey should never be fed to infants. For kids and

---

[47] http://nutritiondata.self.com/facts/fruits-and-fruit-juices/1809/2

[48] http://nutritiondata.self.com/facts/beverages/3873/2

adults choose unpasteurized honey as the pasteurization process removes some of the health benefits.

- **Maple syrup:** Made from the sap of maple trees, organic, pure maple syrup is full of antioxidants, manganese, riboflavin, zinc, magnesium, calcium, and potassium. Similar to honey, darker varieties contain more antioxidants than do lighter syrups.
- **Coconut sugar:** Extracted from the sap of the coconut flower, coconut sugar is rich in polyphenols, iron, zinc, calcium, potassium, antioxidants, phosphorus, and other phytonutrients. It also contains a small amount of fiber called inulin.
- **Organic blackstrap molasses:** Blackstrap molasses is a byproduct of cane sugar's refining process: Cane sugar is mashed to create juice. It's then boiled once to create cane syrup. A second boiling creates molasses. After this syrup has been boiled a third time, a dark, viscous liquid emerges known to Americans as blackstrap molasses. It has the lowest sugar content of any cane sugar product. The unique aspect of blackstrap molasses is that, unlike refined sugar, which has zero nutritional value, blackstrap molasses contains vital vitamins and minerals, such as iron, calcium, magnesium, vitamin B6, and selenium.

Low-Calorie Sweeteners

Low-calorie sweeteners can generally be divided into two categories: artificial and natural. The taste of sweeteners is typically hundreds, even tens of thousands times sweeter than sugar. They are often combined with other products to cover up bitter aftertastes. And all this without any calories? If it seems too good to be true, it probably is. Although most of these products don't actually contain calories, many of them still stimulate receptors in our bodies with downstream consequences, such as insulin resistance.[49]

Even when used in small doses, the effect on taste buds is powerful. The more sweeteners in the diet, the more we train our kids' taste buds to crave sugar, which leads to more sugary snacks, more breads and simple starches, and more processed foods. The whining continues, and the addiction worsens. Also, many of us see low-calorie sweeteners (like Stevia and monk fruit) as "safe" or "not as bad as" sugar, which gives us a false sense of security and allows sugar to infiltrate our foods, lives, and bodies.

Additionally, few low-calorie sweeteners have been subjected to long-term studies, particularly in children, to prove their safe use in food. Some common low-calorie sweeteners are listed in Figure 5.4.

Artificial Low-Calorie Sweeteners	Natural Low-Calorie Sweeteners
Aspartame (Equal)	Stevia (Truvia, Pure Via, Stevia in the Raw)
Advantame	Monk Fruit (Pure Lo)
Neotame (Nutrasweet)	Yacon Syrup
Saccharin (Sweet'N Low)	Allulose
Sucralose (Splenda)	Tagatose
Ace K (Sunett or Sweet One)	
Cyclamate (Sugar Twin)	

Figure 5.4

Stevia and Monk Fruit

Two "natural" low-calorie sweeteners that have become quite popular over the last few years are stevia leaf and monk fruit. The stevia plant (aka sweet leaf or candyleaf) is native to South

49 https://pubmed.ncbi.nlm.nih.gov/30535090/

America. It is two hundred times sweeter than sugar and has become a popular marketing component for "healthier products." But there are many garbage versions of this product out there. Because stevia can have a bitter aftertaste, many products made with it will also include other sweeteners (such as erythritol) to counteract this. Fortunately, stevia does not directly cause weight gain or spikes in insulin. Although it is absorbed, it is quickly eliminated by the liver and kidneys. Thus far, it has not been shown to be carcinogenic.

Unfortunately, it's not all rainbows and unicorns with stevia. If you remember back to Chapter 4 on gut health, our intestinal microbiome is vitally important to our skin and inflammatory level. Stevia has been shown in several studies to have negative effects on our gut bacteria, such as limiting their ability to grow by damaging their environment. Stevia makes our colon less acidic and reduces ammonium levels. In this altered environment, bacteria have difficulty producing short-chain fatty acids (SCFAs), which colon cells use for energy.[50]

Monk fruit is a small, green melon native to Southeast Asia, named for its use by monks in the 1300s. Similar to stevia, it is often combined with sugar alcohols like xylitol or erythritol, thus defeating the purpose of the "natural" product. These additional ingredients can cause stomach upset, vomiting, and diarrhea. Similar to stevia, monk fruit also maintains a low glycemic index (no insulin spike) and does not directly lead to weight gain. No studies currently exist on the interaction of monk fruit sweeteners and our gut bacteria.

50 https://pubmed.ncbi.nlm.nih.gov/31311146/

The Bottom Line

I recommend avoiding low-calorie sweeteners, if possible. If you must use one of these products, the natural sweeteners like stevia or monk fruit are probably the better options at this point, though studies are limited. If using these products, make sure there are no additives or preservatives, avoid liquid versions containing alcohol, and *make sure you count them as added sugar* for the day. I use organic dates, coconut sugar, honey, and maple syrup with a goal to keep added sugar under 24 grams per day.

Avoid liquid versions of natural sweeteners containing alcohol and make sure you count them as added sugar for the day.

Processed Foods

Not only are processed foods packed with sugar, but they are also chock-full of chemicals to provide taste, long-term shelf stability, texture, and colors. The majority of these additives are not found in natural foods, so our bodies see them as foreign. The reactions to these chemicals range from general inflammation to eczema, from negative effects on our nervous system and brain to cancers, and worse. Unfortunately, in the U.S., the food lobby is so powerful that we eat chemicals every day that have been outlawed for years by most European countries.

My personal and professional opinion is that all processed foods should be removed from children's diets. But I'm pragmatic enough to realize that's not always possible in today's world. Below are some of the additives which have been shown by studies to have negative effects on eczema.

- **Sulfur dioxide and other sulfites:** These are used as preservatives in a wide range of foods, especially soft drinks, sausages, burgers, and dried fruits and vegetables. They have been implicated in asthma and eczema, from both ingestion and contact from fruit that has been treated.[51] Be sure to check your food labels—sulfite is often the second word in an ingredient, such as potassium bisulfite.
- **Preservatives butylated hydroxytoluene (BHT) and butylated hydroxyanisole (BHA):** In studying rats given the preservative BHT, researchers found an increase in immediate skin allergies, linking it to an allergic response. BHT caused a type of white blood cell, known as mast cells, to release the chemicals histamine and leukotrienes.[52] These chemicals caused an allergic response in the skin and an eczema-like reaction. Both BHT and BHA have been banned in Europe over concerns of cancer risk.
- **Benzoic acid and other benzoates:** These are used as food preservatives—most commonly in soft drinks—to prevent yeasts and molds from growing. They occur naturally in fruit and honey. Benzoates could make the symptoms of asthma and eczema worse in children who already have these conditions. Additionally, their use in cosmetics may cause contact dermatitis.[53]
- **Tartrazine (yellow food dye) and other azo dyes:** In low chronic doses, food colorings can aggravate the skin. It may not always cause an acute or life-threatening allergic reaction, but it will constantly aggravate *eczema* and make it harder to treat.[54] How can eating a yellow lollipop cause

[51] https://pubmed.ncbi.nlm.nih.gov/24834193/
[52] https://pubmed.ncbi.nlm.nih.gov/17604070/
[53] https://www.ncbi.nlm.nih.gov/pmc/articles/PMC7394164/
[54] https://doi.org/10.1016/j.yrtph.2006.11.004

such problems? Tartrazine stimulates the production of pro-inflammatory leukotrienes.[55] A randomized study in England also found children who ingested food dyes and the preservative sodium benzoate had significant increases in hyperactivity.[56]

With all the sugars and chemicals added to our foods, grocery shopping can be a daunting experience, as families attempt to remove toxins from their diet. I have added The Eczema Pantry at the end of this book to help guide families in purchasing the common pantry staples we use every day. We also include The Eczema Kitchen at the end to provide food substitutions, meal planning, and recipes.

I could write an entire novel on food additives alone. As I attempted to navigate this complicated food world to heal my daughter's skin, I was overwhelmed. It took years of fighting with my husband, in-laws, and even my colleagues to elicit a change in our thinking about food. Fast-forward twelve years: my daughter now has beautiful, eczema-free skin, but it's practically taken years off my life to get us here. In my Eczema Transformation Program, we provide families with brands of foods and snacks, shopping tips and tricks, and recipes to make this transition easier. In the next chapter, we will discuss how I took away my family's favorite drink of all time, and why my husband finally thanked me for it.

Chapter Takeaways

- The United States leads the world in sugar intake. High sugar levels increase inflammation in our bodies, wreak

[55] https://pubmed.ncbi.nlm.nih.gov/11251628/

[56] https://www.sciencedirect.com/science/article/abs/pii/S0140673607613063

havoc on our gut bacteria, and directly affect our skin by binding to skin proteins—all resulting in worsening eczema.

- Sugar has many alternate names and forms that we must consider when counting our daily intake.
- The chemicals—including additives, preservatives, and dyes—in processed foods have been directly linked to worsening allergic diseases, such as eczema and asthma.

In addition to The Eczema Kitchen recipes at the end of the book, additional recipes to reduce sugar can be found at our book resource page by scanning the QR code below.

6

The Problem with Dairy

Breastfeeding is one of the most important things we can do for our babies to help them build healthy guts, decrease childhood disease, increase IQ, and create an emotional bond. Unfortunately, breastfeeding is sometimes not possible because of life circumstances or an issue with mom or baby. Managing the world of baby formulas can be incredibly overwhelming for mothers. Simply managing the world of dairy alternatives for parents of milk-drinking kids can be a struggle as well. Enter 4-month-old Aiden and his frustrated mother, Monica.

I first met Aiden and Monica a few years ago. Aiden had recently developed eczema, and Monica was searching desperately to find help. At about three months of age, Aiden was not gaining weight as he should, and Monica's pediatrician felt that she was simply not producing enough breast milk. Monica was doing everything possible to maintain a healthy lifestyle and felt guilty that she couldn't provide her baby with adequate nutrition.

On the advice of her pediatrician, she had started Aiden on a supplemental baby formula, which, of course, contained dairy, as most do. Within a couple weeks of starting the formula, Aiden began to develop the characteristic red, inflamed, rough patches of eczema on his previously clear, soft skin. As a response to the outbreak, Monica switched to a dairy-free formula for several weeks but saw no improvement. In fact, Aiden's eczema got worse. As a last-ditch effort, she switched back to dairy formula. She chose an organic product, thinking fewer toxins would help, but Aiden's skin continued to deteriorate. When he was one year old, she started him on organic full-fat (whole) milk. But things just kept getting worse, so she decided to change to lactose-free milk to try to "reduce" his dairy exposure.

Monica was desperate, and she blamed herself. As she sat in my office in tears, she explained, "If I could just have made enough breast milk, none of this would have happened. I can't believe I did this to him." Crushing mother guilt had overwhelmed Monica. My heart sank for her. I have a long, complex history with my own mother guilt. You feel solely responsible for these little creatures, and when problems arise it seems that everyone looks to you for the answer.

Does this sound familiar to you? Have you ever had something bad happen to your child, and you felt responsible? Even when it's something you had absolutely no control over, like Monica, you feel guilty.

After giving Monica a great big hug, I began to talk to her about eczema. I explained that the reasons for Aiden's eczema development were much more nuanced than simply a breast milk issue.

As you learned in previous chapters, just being born in the United States drastically increases your chance of contracting eczema. Aiden was also using *teethers*, which are sugar-filled biscuits aimed at soothing painful gums in babies. The last chapter showed us that sugar is a major culprit in eczema.

And finally, there is the problem with dairy, which also happened to be a major problem in my family. Our family drank an absurd amount of milk. We typically would drink a gallon and a half of milk per day, sometimes more. When the kids came in from playing outside, we would quench their thirst with a big glass of cold milk rather than water. Each night, my husband would eat several bowls of cereal before bed (sugar and dairy overload).

We were drinking skim milk because the food industry had tricked us into thinking all fat was bad. Then we shifted to organic whole milk as the first step toward cleaning up our diets, but our inflammatory conditions remained despite the cleaner dairy products. It wasn't until we were forced to remove dairy as part of my daughter's eczema treatment program that we noticed the biggest changes. Her skin rapidly improved, my belly felt better, and my husband noticed his joint pain was better! Now, I am not sure we can chalk all that up to dairy removal, but I definitely think there was a link.

The Devil Is in the Dairy Details

I want to begin by saying that dairy is not the devil. There are some definite benefits to dairy, particularly cow's milk. Milk is naturally packed full of essential vitamins and minerals, like A, B2, B3, B6, B12, magnesium, phosphorus, potassium, zinc, and selenium. Trace amounts of vitamin A, D, E, and K are found in whole milk, although most of these vitamins are added by the manufacturer. Milk is also a great source of fats, proteins, and omega-3s. But I wouldn't have titled this chapter the way I did if there weren't some major drawbacks as well, particularly related to eczema.

When dairy cows became an industrialized asset, everything changed. The pasteurization of milk (which involves boiling it at high temperatures) allows a more shelf-stable product for sale in stores and removes potential foodborne pathogens, but at a cost. Pasteurization alters the fats, proteins, calcium, and oils found in milk. It also destroys the natural (and beneficial) probiotics. These beneficial bacteria are known to help produce lactase, the enzyme needed for humans to digest the milk sugar, lactose. As a result, approximately 68 percent of the world has problems absorbing lactose, and certain ethnicities are disproportionately affected (as evidenced in Figure 6.1).[57]

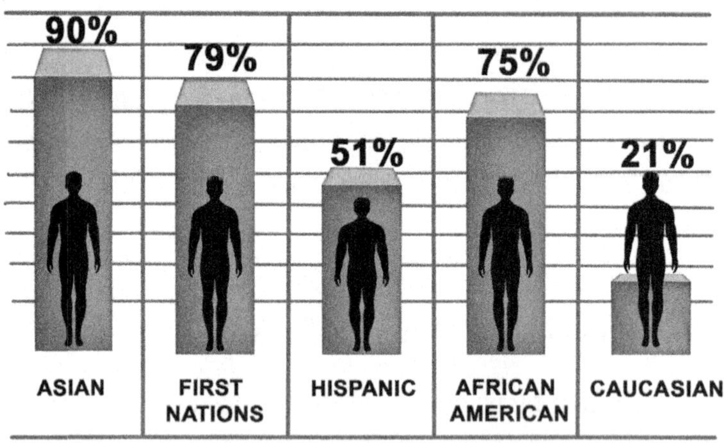

Figure 6.1

With these levels of lactose intolerance, it begs the question: is cow's milk really a great option for humans? To answer this question, we must examine the protein content in milk.

Casein is a protein that accounts for more than 80 percent of the protein in milk. There are several types of casein. Beta-casein (consisting of two variants: A1 and A2) makes up about 30 percent of all the casein in milk. Historically, cows only produced

[57] https://pubmed.ncbi.nlm.nih.gov/28690131/

the A2 type of beta-casein. But due to genetic mutations over many thousands of years, the milk sold in stores today (particularly in Western countries) primarily contains the A1 variant.

When A1 milk is digested in the small intestine, it produces a peptide called beta-casomorphin-7 (BCM-7). The intestines absorb BCM-7, and it passes into the blood. Doctors have linked BCM-7 to stomach discomfort and symptoms similar to those experienced by people with lactose intolerance. Additionally, the movement of BCM-7 into the blood via a leaky gut has been implicated in the development of type 1 diabetes, coronary artery disease, and even autism, particularly if immune deficiencies are present.[58]

Cow's Milk Protein Allergy (CMPA)

Cow's milk protein allergy (CMPA) is the most common food allergy in patients with eczema. It typically starts in the first year of life. As we discussed in our food allergy testing chapter, there are typically two types of problems with cow's milk protein: acute *allergy* and *sensitivity*. True acute CMPA (less common) shows severe symptoms immediately upon ingesting and shows up during classic milk allergy testing.

Milk protein *sensitivity* is much more common, yet subtle, as it can take up to nine days after ingestion to show symptoms. Additionally, this is NOT tested during a typical milk allergy test. Thus, you may be having a reaction to milk/dairy despite a negative milk allergy test. For all these reasons, dairy is one of the first eliminations we recommend for patients suffering from eczema. And because there can be cross-reactivity between different

---

58 https://www.ncbi.nlm.nih.gov/pmc/articles/PMC8345738/

animal milk sources, I also initially recommend removing goat, sheep, and camel milk products.

The Dairy Solution

Inevitably, as soon as I make this recommendation, a number of questions arise:

- What about calcium?
- What about vitamin D?
- How do we understand milk labels for nutrients and ingredients?
- Which milk substitutes are best?
- Does this mean my child will never have dairy again?

As kids, many of us are encouraged to drink lots of milk because "we need calcium for strong bones." While calcium is important for the growing child, milk is definitely not the only reliable source, despite what the milk industry has been saying for years. In fact, there is no conclusive evidence to show that drinking milk actually strengthens our bones.[59] Additionally, whole milk contains only trace amounts of vitamin D, and most of that is added by the dairy processor.

The recommended daily intake of calcium varies widely from country to country. The United States recommends higher intake than most countries, as seen in Figure 6.2 (next page). However, the U.S. recommendations are based on short-term studies from the 1970s that have never been replicated, raising concerns over their validity. The higher recommended intake has not lowered the risk of fractures or osteoporosis in the U.S. More evidence continues to emerge that vitamin D plays a larger role in bone health than calcium.

---

[59] https://jamanetwork.com/journals/jamapediatrics/fullarticle/1769138

The recommended intakes for calcium in the United Kingdom (and most other countries) are significantly lower, as shown in Figure 6.2. I recommend meeting the U.K. standards as your daily minimum requirement.

Recommended Daily Calcium Intake By Country		
Age	**United States/Canada**	**United Kingdom**
0–6 months	200mg	525mg
6–12 months	260mg	525mg
1–3 years	700mg	350mg
4–6 years	1000mg	450mg
6–8 years	1000mg	550mg
9–10 years (female)	1300mg	550mg
9–10 years (male)	1300mg	550mg
11–18 years (female)	1300mg	800mg
11–18 years (male)	1300mg	1000mg
19–50 years	1000mg	700mg
51–70 years (female)	1200mg	700mg
51–70 years (male)	1000mg	700mg
71+	1200mg	700mg

https://www.bda.uk.com/resource/calcium.html [60, 61, 62]

Figure 6.2

Let's look at milk by the numbers. One cup of milk typically provides about 276 mg of calcium. However, there are many

60 https://ods.od.nih.gov/factsheets/Calcium-HealthProfessional/

61 https://www.bda.uk.com/resource/calcium.html

62 https://www.canada.ca/en/health-canada/services/food-nutrition/healthy-eating/vitamins-minerals/vitamin-calcium-updated-dietary-reference-intakes-nutrition.html

non-dairy foods with high calcium content. Figure 6.3 shows non-dairy foods rich in calcium. In my Eczema Transformation Program, I provide more extensive lists of calcium-rich foods and recipes to incorporate into your child's diet. In addition, my health coach addresses this issue regularly in our weekly live group meetings, so you can personalize the advice to your family's needs.

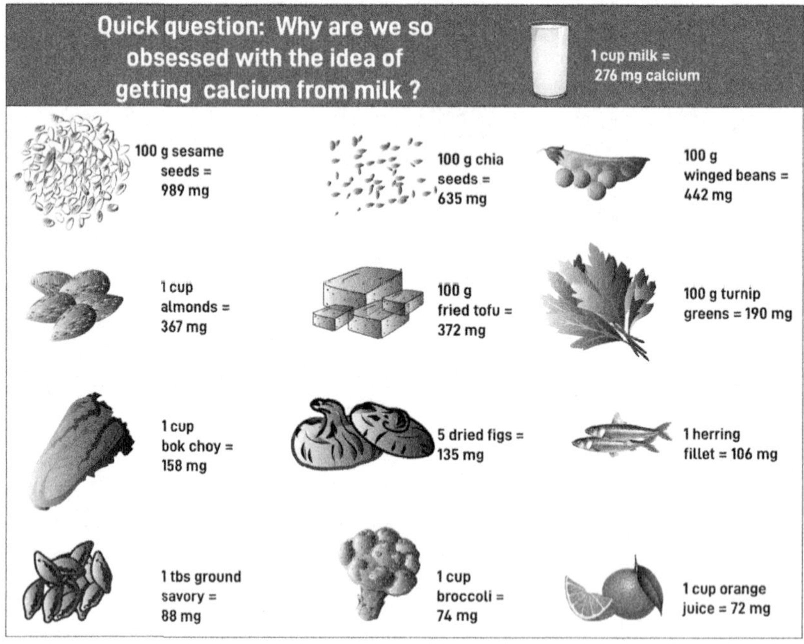

Figure 6.3

As you can see, there are a lot of other great ways to add calcium to your diet, so don't let the calcium ogres scare you. A fast and easy way to determine the calcium content in a product is to check the label for the percentage of calcium and replace the % with a zero. So, if the serving has "45% calcium," that equates to 450 mg of calcium per serving.

Non-Dairy Milk Alternatives

There are a number of non-dairy milk alternatives on the market these days, and more coming weekly. Plant-based milks vary quite a bit in their ingredients and flavor. My general rule is to look at the label of ingredients—if it contains numerous fillers and natural flavors (i.e., words that end with *ite*, *ate*, or *ide*), then typically I move on. Many brands are fortified with calcium and vitamin D but use a number of additives to include these nutrients. I recommend buying a cleaner plant-based milk and incorporating vitamin D and calcium from other whole foods or from clean supplements. (We will discuss vitamin D in more detail in Chapter 9.)

Here are some comparisons of common plant-based milks on the market.

Non-Dairy Milk Alternatives: How Do They Compare?

Nutrition facts information for cow's milk and fortified, unsweetened non-dairy milk alternatives per one cup (240mL) serving

	Cow's milk	Almond	Coconut Carton	Coconut full-fat, canned	Hemp	Oat	Rice	Soy
Calories and Macronutrients								
Calories (kcal)	120	30	40	420	80	60	70	80
Carbohydrates (g)	12	1	1	6	1	7	11	3
Total fat (g)	5	2.5	4	45	8	3	2.5	4
Protein (g)	8	1	0	1	2	1	0	7
Micronutrients (% daily value)								
Calcium	29%	35%	35%	0%	30%	35%	25%	20%
Vitamin D	26%	25%	10%	0%	25%	15%	25%	15%

The information provided in this table is based on nutrition facts information provided by manufacturers of various commercially available beverages. Nutritional information varies depending on the brand, flavor, added vitamins and minerals, and ingredients.

Figure 6.4
Note: the non-dairy alternatives above are typically fortified with calcium and vitamin D and vary by brand. Be sure to check the label on your specific brand.

> If you are interested in making your own non-dairy milk, be sure to check out The Eczema Kitchen in the back of the book for recipes.

Now, back to Monica and Aiden. I did a thorough review of Aiden's diet.

- Breakfast: cereal with lactose-free milk
- Lunch: sandwich with ham/cheese, Go-Gurt, pretzels, grapes

- Snack: Cheese-Its, Goldfish crackers, pretzels
- Dinner: macaroni and cheese, pasta with butter, or chicken and rice

What I noticed, aside from a glaring lack of plants, is dairy overload. Monica and I discussed Aiden's dairy sources: butter, milk, yogurt, cheese, ice cream—not to mention dairy in packaged products like Cheez-Its and Goldfish. I put together a plan to temporarily replace dairy in the entire family's diet while we healed Aiden's gut. (I also include a number of dairy alternatives in The Eczema Pantry at the end of this book.)

You may ask, "What? The whole family? Why?" It is exceptionally difficult to do an elimination diet for one child. The child feels persecuted, less loved, and lesser than the rest of the family. When the whole family eats the same foods, whining decreases, food struggles lessen, and the path to healing is much faster. Plus, since the whole family has a similar microbiome, if one person in the family has a dairy issue, most of the other members likely have a similar issue. It does not mean everyone has eczema; some members may have belly issues, such as reflux or high cholesterol, or some may have joint pains or acne. The root cause is the same: inflammation from dairy.

When the whole family eats the same foods, whining decreases, food struggles lessen, and the path to healing is much faster.

In my clinic and my online eczema transformation course, when families work together toward the goal of clear skin, improvement is seen faster and flares recur less often. Not to mention, the stress in the home is significantly reduced. Moms have lost weight, gained more energy, and experienced less reflux, while dads have seen improvement in their seasonal allergies, headaches, and cholesterol levels. But don't just take my word—check out what moms and dads have to say about our program by scanning the QR code at the end of this chapter.

Monica and her husband did an amazing job of getting on the same page to temporarily replace dairy. Over several weeks, they watched their son's skin begin to heal. Of course, that's not the whole story—we had to do more than just food replacement, as you will see in the next several chapters.

For Aiden, limiting processed foods and sugar and temporarily removing dairy made a huge difference. But what if you have already done this and the skin shows zero improvement? Join me in the next chapter, where we will examine a pesky protein that has taken over our diets and left many people with out-of-control inflammation.

Chapter Takeaways

- A large portion of the world is lactose intolerant. Changes in the way milk is processed have led to additional systemic inflammation from milk proteins.
- Cow's milk protein allergy (CMPA) is the most common food allergy in patients with eczema. It typically starts in the first year of life.

- Non-dairy milk alternatives are a viable replacement for cow's milk and calcium, though be sure to check for added fillers or flavors, which may cause inflammation.

In addition to The Eczema Kitchen recipes at the end of the book, additional recipes to replace dairy can be found at our book resource page by scanning the QR code below.

7

The Gluten Conundrum

I remember sitting in a restaurant with my husband about fifteen years ago. We were rolling our eyes and making snarky comments about the lady next to us, as she tortured the server talking about her numerous food sensitivities and concerns. "I need to make sure the chef understands that I cannot have any dairy, and I want to avoid gluten as well. Could you please confirm with the kitchen that none of these products will be served in my meal?" the lady pleaded. My husband and I even joked about her on the plane on the way home. "Can you believe that crazy lady with all the food issues? Man, imagine living with her!"

Oh, how far we have come. That crazy lady is now me.

I experienced my personal reckoning with gluten about eight years ago. I had suffered from stomach issues for as long as I could remember. Two of my most favorite things in the world were bread and beer, although I had to take Miralax ***every day for twenty-five years*** to help me poop. I dealt with stomach bloating and pain daily, but I never associated my belly issues with a particular food.

I had to take Miralax *every day for twenty-five years* to help me poop.

My *Aha* moment came when I was prepping for a tropical vacation and chose to take a tiny bikini I was hoping to get into. The problem was, the mini bikini in question looked awful with my bloated belly. So, my grand idea was to abstain from beer and bread while on vacation for the sole purpose of looking good in my bathing suit. Two weeks later, upon arriving home, I noted that my daily belly pain had resolved and there was no more bloating.

I decided to give it a few more weeks, although I was definitely craving bread. After a month, I no longer needed Miralax daily. My life was changed from that point onward. So, yes, vanity is initially what drove me away from gluten. But the following patient experience is what inspired me to tell others to do the same.

A Lesson in Gluten

I met Jada when she was less than two years old. She was a rambunctious toddler without a care in the world, brought in by her mother, Amanda, because of worsening eczema and allergies. According to Amanda, Jada had started developing eczema symptoms about six months prior, but also was having recurrent ear infections and a runny nose. Upon further questioning, there was a distant relative with celiac disease, but Jada had not shown any GI issues whatsoever. Jada had actually seen my colleague first, who had referred her for lab testing to screen for celiac disease. Those results had come back negative, and my colleague had told Amanda, "This is definitely NOT gluten-related, as her labs are negative and she has no GI symptoms."

But Amanda confided in me that she had kept Jada off gluten for a few weeks and some of her symptoms had seemed to improve. I had a chat with my colleague about Jada's case, and I will never forget his response: "Why would you restrict a child from eating tasty food like Burger King and Goldfish crackers without definitive evidence of celiac disease? I mean, these are the foods that make childhood fun."

At the time, I didn't have the full body response that I now get when thinking about his comments. I was thinking about my own gluten experience and the fact that Amanda had noted some improvement in Jada's skin and runny nose while off gluten. With this in mind, I formulated a plan with Amanda to keep her off gluten for a 3-month trial.

When Jada returned after three months, Amanda was all smiles. Jada's eczema had mostly cleared, and there had been no runny nose and no ear infections since the last visit. So Amanda and I decided to try a gluten reintroduction so that Jada wouldn't have to miss out on "fun kid food." (I no longer believe in the "fun kid food" concept. Feeding kids crap simply because it tastes good makes no sense to me.)

Fast-forward another three months to Jada's next follow-up. I asked Amanda about the gluten reintroduction and if Jada had any recurrent symptoms. "Well, the gluten reintroduction was interesting. We started back with some bread products and within 48 hours Jada was having toddler tantrums like never before. I didn't think it could be gluten-related because it was all behavioral. But after another two weeks of inconsolable tantrums at home and at daycare, I decided to remove gluten again. And just like that, her behavior returned to normal."

I didn't know how to respond. I just didn't have enough gluten experience under my belt to make heads or tails of what Amanda was telling me. I just knew there must be more to this gluten story than traditional medicine was willing to admit at the time (and still is). I recommended Jada stay off gluten until we healed her gut, despite my ignorance as to why her behavior worsened from its reintroduction. But now I was on a mission to figure out this problem. Many more questions arose in my head.

- Are any of my other patients suffering from a gluten issue that is not classic celiac disease?
- Could gluten be causing issues other than just abdominal bloating and pain, like I had experienced?
- Could some food or medication be negatively affecting a child, although traditional medicine said it wasn't?

I knew I needed to do some serious research and fieldwork on gluten. Here is what I have found over the last eight years.

Gluten Unraveled

Gluten (from the Latin *glutin*, meaning glue) is a group of proteins found in wheat, barley, and rye. They act like glue by helping foods bind together. Gluten is added to many other foods as a binding agent to help the consistency of the food itself. (Gluten is what makes pizza dough stretchy, for example.) Issues with gluten can range from gluten intolerance (celiac disease) to a sensitivity, as we discussed in Chapter 2.

Celiac disease carries a genetic component and is diagnosed by blood testing or by biopsy of the small intestine. Patients have an immune response to gluten, leading to bloating, diarrhea, gas, fatigue, anemia, and other symptoms. Lifelong health consequences—including cardiac disease, thyroid issues, and cancers—can be seen with untreated celiac disease. Approximately 1 in 100 people are affected by celiac disease.

A second group of patients has emerged. They have very similar symptoms to celiac disease but have a negative blood test and negative biopsy findings. Despite the negative testing, when these patients are given a gluten-free diet, their symptoms resolve in a similar fashion to those of celiac patients. This condition, called non-celiac gluten sensitivity (NCGS), is the much more controversial younger brother of celiac disease and has a more complex connection to health issues. It is estimated that up to 13 percent of the population may exhibit NCGS, although many of these studies cite self-reported cases.[63]

Furthermore, it remains unclear whether the true culprit in NCGS is the gluten itself, the wheat, or the pesticides used in production of the wheat.[64] To better understand, we need to look back at the history of wheat.

The Early Days of Wheat

Ancient wheat species (e.g., einkorn, spelt, and emmer) were all "covered" grains, characterized by having thick husks around each seed. The inedible husk (also known as the chaff) had to be removed via a labor-intensive process (threshing and winnowing) before wheat could be used in food preparation, hence the idiom "separate the wheat from the chaff" to describe separating things that are higher in quality.

Today's modern wheat is considered to be a "naked wheat" cultivar, with a much thinner husk that is easy to remove. A number of other changes have occurred in the cultivation of wheat, leading to what we now call hybridized wheat.

Over the past several hundred years, humans have learned how to improve crop characteristics to increase yields. Owing to the work of Gregor Mendel, the monk who learned how to genetically manipulate pea plants, wheat growers began to modify the plants to grow larger seeds and smaller stalks. Ancient wheat varieties were over 6 feet tall and had small seeds, while modern

63 https://www.ncbi.nlm.nih.gov/pmc/articles/PMC6182669/
64 https://www.ncbi.nlm.nih.gov/pmc/articles/PMC7762999/

versions are 2–3 feet tall with comparatively massive seeds (see Figure 7.1). The shorter plants were also modified to hold their seeds, and to become tolerant of nitrogen-heavy fertilizer, herbicides, and pesticides. By redirecting most of the wheat plant's energy toward the seeds and higher yields, an unintended result was a wheat plant with drastically higher levels of gluten.

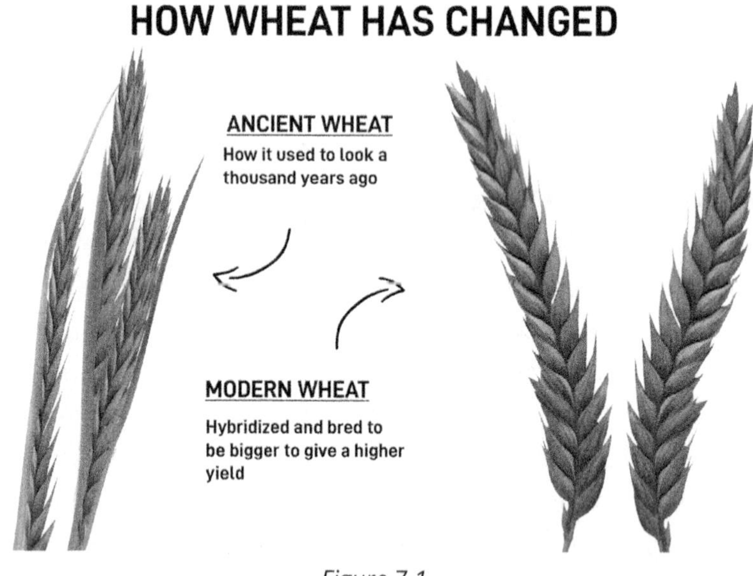

Figure 7.1

The Roundup on Wheat

The next wrinkle in the gluten conundrum concerns the chemicals that are used to grow modern wheat. Farmers spray wheat fields with a chemical pesticide called glyphosate (commonly known as Roundup) to kill weeds. Additional glyphosate is applied just before harvest, as it speeds the drying of the wheat for processing and allows easier removal of the seeds. Thus, most harvested wheat has high levels of fresh pesticide. A great amount of controversy exists over the question of what, exactly, is causing the dramatic increase in gluten sensitivity: glyphosate, or the gluten itself? The incidence of gluten sensitivity has risen steadily alongside the use of glyphosate on crops (see Figure 7.2).[65]

Celiac Incidence and Glyphosate Use

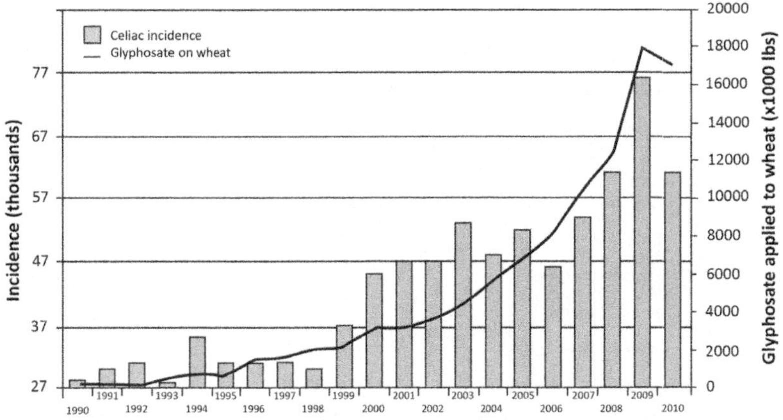

Image Courtesy of Samsel and Seneff, Interdiscip Toxicol.2013;6(4):159-184

Figure 7.2

Glyphosate is known to wreak havoc on the bacteria in our guts, while the resulting inflammation can damage the intestinal wall. It's also important to note that glyphosate has been determined to be carcinogenic. Monsanto (now owned by Bayer) has been forced by numerous lawsuits to pay millions of dollars for causing cancer.[66]

The Environmental Working Group (EWG) routinely tests consumer items and foods for harmful substances. EWG tested popular breakfast cereals for glyphosate levels, with disturbing findings. Ironically, that healthy attempt at "low sugar" oat

---

65 https://www.ncbi.nlm.nih.gov/pmc/articles/PMC3945755/

66 https://www.npr.org/2020/06/24/882949098/bayer-to-pay-more-than-10-billion-to-resolve-roundup-cancer-lawsuits

cereal may just have given you a whopping dose of pesticide (see Figure 7.3). Although I consider *any* glyphosate harmful, the EWG sets their threshold at 160 parts per billion (ppb).

Results Of EWG's 2018 Glyphosate Tests In Oat Breakfast Cereals

Type of Product	Product Name	Glyphosate (ppb)			Lab
		Sample 1	Sample 2	Sample 3	
Oat Breakfast Cereal	Barbara's Multigrain Spoonfuls, Cereal Original	340	300		Eurofins
	Apple Cinnamon Cheerios	868			Anresco
	Cheerios Oat Crunch Cinnamon	1171	541		Anresco
	Cheerios Toasted Whole Grain Oat Cereal	490	470	530	Eurofins
	Chocolate Cheerios	826			Anresco
	Frosted Cheerios	756	893		Anresco
	Fruity Cheerios	618			Anresco
	Honey Nut Cheerios	833	894		Anresco
	Very Berry Cheerios	810			Anresco
	Kellogg's Cracklin' Oat Bran	250	120		Eurofins
	Lucky Charms	400	230		Eurofins
	Quaker Oatmeal Squares Brown Sugar	2746			Anresco
	Quaker Oatmeal Squares Honey Nut	2837			Anresco
	Kashi Heart to Heart Organic Honey Toasted	ND	ND		Eurofins

Figure 7.3

The Bread and Butter of Breadmaking

Not only has the way we *grow* wheat changed over time, the way we *prepare* wheat has also changed significantly. Let's look at the history of breadmaking to understand the connection.

The invention of quick-rise commercial yeasts in the 1950s fundamentally altered the way we've baked bread since ancient times. The traditional way to make bread is very similar to the way we currently make sourdough bread. Sourdough has been a kind friend to our guts through the ages, for one primary reason—it's easier to digest. Before the quick-rise commercial yeast, or "baker's yeast," was popularized in the 1950s and '60s, we made bread with a sourdough starter. It's a mix of fermented grain and water, which collects the wild yeast that lives all around us in the air, on our bodies, and in the flour itself.

The complex, symbiotic ecosystem of a sourdough starter works to leaven, flavor, and build the structure of the dough. The slow fermentation process invites a magical combination of wild yeast, bacteria, enzymes, and *lactobacillus* (the same bacteria in yogurt) to release lactic acid and create the sour flavor that sourdough is known for. The enzymes unlock minerals in the wheat that are otherwise unavailable to us. The yeast, which feeds on complex starches, releases carbon dioxide as a byproduct. Gluten traps the carbon dioxide and creates the rise and texture of the loaf.[67]

The longer the dough ferments, the more the gluten is broken down for us. Of course, our ancestors knew this, to some degree. The magic of baking bread was understood long before we learned the science of it.

Sourdough uses a process called *hydrolysis*, in which enzymes break down large, indigestible proteins into smaller amino acids. A number of these indigestible proteins, such as fructan and phytic acid, have been implicated as part of gluten sensitivity.

Several recent studies point to fructan, a compound found in bread and other things like bananas and garlic, as the source of gluten sensitivity. Many gluten-sensitive people have found digestive relief from avoiding foods with fructan (aka FODMAPS).[68] Sourdough bread does not contain fructan once it goes through fermentation. Other studies point to phytic acid, an acid found in

---

67 https://www.huffpost.com/entry/sourdough-bread-gluten-celiac_n_5b213232e4b0adfb82702959

68 https://www.huffpost.com/entry/sourdough-bread-gluten-celiac_n_5b213232e4b0adfb82702959

wheat flour that breaks down during sourdough fermentation, as a contributor to gluten sensitivity.[69]

The components of bread that are hypothesized to be toxic to gluten-sensitive people are typically rendered digestible during sourdough fermentation. Our modern, white, starchy breads don't see the benefit of this natural fermentation, and the resulting digestion difficulty may be related to gluten sensitivity.

Breads and pastas aren't the only source of gluten. As mentioned earlier, it is a binding agent for foods. To improve the consistency of foods or sauces, food companies will typically add vital gluten, which is a specialized flour that has been processed to contain high concentrations of gluten. Due to this added flour, many foods in the American diet such as soups and dressings are packed with gluten. This fact surprises many people.

So let me say this: *gluten in itself is NOT bad*. The problem lies in how gluten crops are raised and harvested, how gluten-containing products are created, and *the sheer amount of gluten* in our diet. Many Americans are taking in high concentrations of gluten at each meal, possibly overwhelming our gut's ability to process the protein. Even after you cut out notorious gluten-rich foods, there are many hidden sources of gluten you wouldn't even consider.

> *So let me say this—gluten in itself is not bad ... it's the sheer amount.*

[69] https://pubmed.ncbi.nlm.nih.gov/15631515/

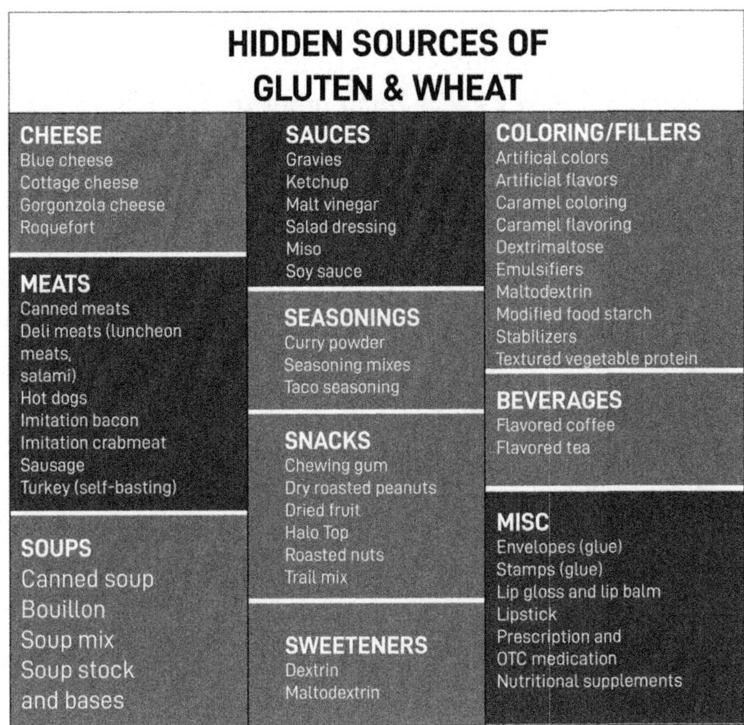

Figure 7.4

I would like to elaborate on a few of the more common culprits.

- **Cereals:** Corn flakes would seem to be a safe choice; as the name implies, they are made from corn. However, most corn flake cereals use malt extract or flavoring, which contain gluten. Of note, any food containing malt likely contains gluten.
- **Granola:** Although granola is typically made from oats, the majority of oat crops are contaminated with gluten because of their close growth proximity to wheat. Unless the oat crop is specifically labeled *gluten-free*, it likely contains gluten.

- **Soy sauce:** Most traditional soy sauces, with the exception of tamari, contain wheat products. Most restaurants offer gluten-free soy sauce upon request.
- **Cream sauces:** To make cream, you typically start with a roux. A roux, composed of equal parts flour and butter, forms the base of the sauce and helps it thicken. Most people use simple, all-purpose flour to make the roux. So, even though your homemade mac and cheese may have gluten-free macaroni, the cheese sauce may very well contain gluten.
- **Chips:** Some potato chip seasonings contain malt vinegar or wheat starch. Most multigrain chips contain gluten unless otherwise listed. Some corn tortilla chips also contain wheat flour. Most crackers and pretzels contain gluten.
- **Soups:** Many soups contain barley, a grain that will add gluten to your bowl. And the Celiac Disease Foundation warns us to "pay special attention to cream-based soups, which have flour as a thickener."[70]
- **Salad dressings and marinades:** Salad sounds safe (at least, if you leave off the croutons). Salad greens don't contain gluten, after all. But you need to think carefully about what you use to top your salad with. Salad dressings routinely contain all kinds of gluten sources. Some incorporate malt vinegar. Others use soy sauce. And still others use flour as a thickener.
- **Meat substitutes:** Many popular meat substitutes—including veggie burgers, vegetarian sausage, imitation bacon, and imitation seafood—are made with seitan.

[70] https://celiac.org/gluten-free-living/gluten-free-foods/

Seitan is actually wheat gluten—exactly what you're trying to avoid.

- **Natural flavor, natural flavoring, and flavoring:** When you see these terms on a label, beware! They may be derived from gluten-containing grains. You will want to investigate further when you see these.
- **Other foods to be aware of:** Brown rice syrup, ice creams, frozen yogurts, lunchmeat, seasoning packets, broth, and boullion.

Given the complexity of the gluten sensitivity problem, I feel the best way to determine whether gluten is contributing to your eczema is to try an elimination/replacement diet. I have been amazed in my practice at how many patients improve dramatically after replacing this one substance. It is difficult, however, given the sheer amount of gluten in so many foods. Fortunately, many restaurants are now aware of gluten sensitivity, and many even have an entire gluten-free menu.

In The Eczema Pantry and Eczema Kitchen at the end of this book, I reference dozens of gluten-free options and substitutes to help you navigate this elimination. My online Eczema Transformation Program helps families coordinate all the issues related to food eliminations, replacements, and reintroduction. Because this topic is so confusing and stressful, my health coach, Lindsay, does group visits once a week to answer questions live, and our families in the community help one another with tips and tricks that have worked for them. It truly takes a village.

The Gluten Stigma

Unfortunately, the term *gluten* is a highly controversial one. It still causes eye rolls in many circles. But I look back on Jada's case and take solace. Although our program reintroduces some gluten after gut healing, Amanda decided to keep Jada permanently gluten-free, and she has thrived. So now, when I hear someone in a restaurant requesting specific ingredients for their food, I think of Jada and how different her life would be if we hadn't decided to act.

We definitely need to understand more about gluten sensitivity and how it affects not only skin but the inflammatory bucket as a whole. In the next chapter, we will discuss another major inflammatory factor that may be affecting your child's skin: histamines.

Chapter Takeaways

- Gluten sensitivity, a less severe form of gluten allergy than celiac disease, has become a recognized source of inflammation for many people with eczema.
- Controversy exists over whether gluten, breakdown products of gluten (including fructan and phytic acid), or the pesticide glyphosate is ultimately responsible for the link between gluten and eczema.
- Changes in the way wheat is grown and prepared, in addition to the many sources of hidden gluten in common

foods, have dramatically increased the amount of gluten in our diets.

In addition to The Eczema Kitchen recipes at the end of the book, more recipes to reduce gluten can be found at our book resource page by scanning the QR code below.

8

Histamines

During the 18 months I lived and practiced in New Zealand, I saw dozens of diseases that I had only read about in books. From rare genetic disorders that occur in the Maori people of New Zealand to an actual case of leprosy, I learned to be on the look-out for the odd and unexpected. Such was the case when I met Oliver, a 5-year-old boy with an interesting problem. According to Oliver's mother, any time he ate something, his face turned red, hives developed around his mouth, and he experienced severe belly pain. He was losing weight rapidly, so his primary care doctor had referred him to a "pediatric specialist" to figure out the problem.

In New Zealand, pediatricians are considered specialist consultants, not primary care doctors. I felt immense pressure every day as I attempted to treat incredibly complex cases that had been referred to our clinic. On the day in question, I sent the resident-in-training into the room first, to get Oliver's full history and to buy me some time to research his symptoms. (Yes, doctors Google stuff before we walk into the room.)

Unfortunately, Dr. Google had no insight into the case, so I waited for the resident to give me the scoop. She returned after about 20 minutes and began to present Oliver's case, with trepidation. "For the last year, Oliver has developed worsening eczema. He now has eczema from head to toe and is pretty darn miserable. The parents have no idea what is causing it. He had been to an allergy specialist who just kept increasing his doses of steroids without success. He also complains of frequent abdominal pain," the resident explained.

Before his eczema issues began, Oliver was a happy-go-lucky kid with clear skin and no GI problems. Oliver's previous doctors felt that his was simply a severe case of eczema and that a high dose of steroids should knock it down. The resident then tallied the alarming amount of steroids he had been taking.

At this point, I had no idea what was going on with Oliver, so I stepped into the room and introduced myself. The first thing I noticed was how thin Oliver was. This was a kid who clearly was not eating well. Oliver's mom said, "I really hope you can help him. I am not sure what else to do. No matter how much medication we give him, his skin just doesn't seem to improve. I don't think he is eating because he is so miserable from the eczema."

I was at a loss. Oliver had one of the worst eczema cases I had ever seen and had not responded to any treatments thus far. His eczema truly reached from head to toe, with numerous areas that were open and bleeding. After extensive questioning about Oliver's development, birth history, family and social history, and dietary habits, I left the room to ponder his case.

Histamine Hysteria

If you have ever been stung by a bee or other insect, you have likely experienced a histamine-related response. Google any common inflammatory condition, and you are bound to see numerous attributions to histamines. Antihistamines (Benadryl,

Zyrtec, Claritin, and so on) can be found in abundance in grocery stores and in most people's medicine cabinets (even my dog takes it). But what the heck is it? And if histamine is a normal part of our physiology, why are we continually trying to block it?

To understand, we need to take another trip down the wormhole of our immune system. Keep in mind, it evolved at a time when food exploration was in its infancy and eating the wrong berry or plant could lead to death in the absence of an efficient defense mechanism.

Enter the mast cell—possibly the most badass defender in our immune system's arsenal. The mast cell is basically a roaming piñata, waiting to be smashed open by the stick-wielding, blindfolded kid at the party. Except in this case, it is filled with histamine rather than candy. And rather than a stick-wielding kid releasing the histamine, a food, chemical, pollen, or other substance causes the massive release of the potent histamine chemical.

So, why such a dramatic response?

Each time our body encounters a new or foreign substance, it must decide whether the newcomer is friend or foe. In Chapter 2's discussion on food allergy, an elaborate chain of events in our immune system helps make this determination. But in the case of eczema and many other inflammatory-driven diseases (e.g., asthma, hay fever, ADHD, and food allergy), the immune system begins to overreact to substances that should be considered friendly. The type of antibody our immune system makes is determined by how big of a threat it is deemed. The most threatening invaders will warrant the production of an antibody known as IgE. Once a substance or food has an IgE antibody formed against it, it's as though that invader has "most wanted" posters all over our body.

Mast cells then roam around our tissues and bloodstream, searching for IgE activators. And when it finds one—kapow! It releases its entire load of histamine on the spot. The released histamines start a chain reaction that puts the immune system in overdrive. The most severe form of this reaction is known as anaphylaxis. This is the type of reaction that, if not treated with an emergency shot of epinephrine (the EpiPen) shortly after exposure, can be fatal.

Histamine History

Histamine was first discovered in the early 20th century. Research into histamine has received two Nobel Prizes and has helped to determine the effects of histamine on different tissues.[71]

- In the nose, eyes, and throat, it causes snot and sneezing, with itchy eyes during pollen season.
- In the GI system, histamines cause the production of stomach acid. Because of this, reflux medications like Zantac are actually antihistamines.
- In blood vessels, it causes dilation and leaky walls, allowing other inflammatory cells to move into tissues such as the skin. (Hello, eczema!)
- In the lungs, it causes the airway pipes to tighten (bronchoconstriction), which leads to breathing difficulty.
- In the brain, histamines cause stimulation and alertness, which is why antihistamines often cause drowsiness as a side effect. In contrast, too much histamine in the brain can lead to headaches, brain fog, memory issues, motor

[71] https://www.ncbi.nlm.nih.gov/pmc/articles/PMC7463562/

tics, and irritability. Interestingly, histamine abnormalities have even been implicated in schizophrenia.[72]

- There are likely thousands more actions of histamines that have yet to be discovered.

For eczema sufferers, we will focus on histamines and the skin. When a child already has an overload of histamines, and then eats a food or encounters a substance that releases even more mast cells, the histamine reaction is often manifested in the skin. As capillaries leak and allow the white blood cells into the skin, itching, redness, swelling, and ulceration can occur. But histamines are just one branch of the inflammatory tree. The entire immune system is typically playing a role in the eczema condition.

The next question is: why are kids developing potent IgE antibodies against harmless substances like peanuts or pollen? Although poorly understood, it is likely from an overactive immune system, a leaky gut, and possibly even our traditional treatments. Various factors can influence the baseline amount of circulating histamine, including diet, stress, environment, nutritional deficiencies, drugs, and hormones. As overall histamine load in the body increases, so do the effects seen by progressive, increasing amounts of inflammation—and ultimately anaphylaxis, if left unchecked. In the case of seasonal allergies or eczema, though pollen may be the substance that takes the body into full allergic reaction, it has already been primed by high levels of histamines from the numerous factors listed above.

---

[72] https://www.ncbi.nlm.nih.gov/pmc/articles/PMC8317266/

DAO Deficiency

Once histamine is circulating or in excess, it is cleaned up by an enzyme called diamine oxidase (DAO). DAO is produced in the kidneys, thymus, and by our gut lining—reinforcing the concept that our gut plays an integral role in the development and persistence of eczema. The leaky gut allows large immune-activating molecules to slip through, increasing the immune response and subsequently increasing histamine levels.

Normally, our bodies would respond by producing more DAO to clean up the excess histamine. However, in a sick gut, cells do not produce enough DAO enzyme to deal with all the circulating histamine, so the vicious cycle continues. We also know that certain bacteria produce histamines, further compounding the problem. By disrupting our gut microbiome, we may also be allowing histamine-producing bacteria to win out over our normal gut flora.

I want to re-emphasize that histamines are only one part of the eczema equation, and in my experience, it's not the place to start from a treatment perspective. However, in patients who fail to improve with the typical approaches we have outlined so far, I will tackle histamines as a possible culprit.

When battling histamine overload, there are really two approaches: block the histamine release and response, or reduce the amount of histamine present in the body.

Conventional modern medicine has focused on pharmaceutically blocking the histamine release and response. The power of Big Pharma explains why everyone has heard of Allegra and Zyrtec but few people can tell you what foods are high in histamines. Integrative medicine takes the approach of root cause analysis—investigating what foods or environmental factors are leading to the overload of histamines and addressing those exposures. But that takes longer than a 10-minute appointment.

Histamines are an important part of our physiology. Simply blocking their effects with stronger and stronger medications is a disastrous plan. We can't keep medicating every problem. Americans filled a record 6.3 billion prescriptions in 2020—an average of over *nineteen prescriptions per person!*[73]

Additionally, medications have side effects. For example, using antihistamines such as Zantac to control reflux has been clearly shown to INCREASE eczema development when given to babies and children.[74] The same risk increase has been found with Tylenol dosing in children.[75] We are simply taking sick kids and turning them into sick adults.

Note: Antihistamines can be useful during the initial treatment of eczema. I use antihistamine medication to help simmer down the overactive mast cells, which decreases itching and scratching and, in turn, calms the nerves and helps families cope. But antihistamine use is temporary while I work to heal the gut and skin. Many practitioners tell families their child will be on antihistamines permanently, without looking for the root cause of histamine overload.

Antihistamines can be useful during the initial treatment of eczema.

[73] https://www.statista.com/statistics/238702/us-total-medical-prescriptions-issued/

[74] https://www.ncbi.nlm.nih.gov/pmc/articles/PMC6137535/

[75] https://pubmed.ncbi.nlm.nih.gov/30991122/

Lower Your Histamine Burden

The reality is, we can never rid ourselves of all histamine-producing things. The goal is to lower the overall histamine burden. The first place to start histamine reduction is in the kitchen—the same place where the most meaningful changes to our health occur. (I know, I sound like a broken record.) There are foods that contain high levels of histamine, and there are foods that are more likely to cause the release of preexisting histamine from mast cells. There are also foods that may block the DAO enzyme, resulting in more circulating histamine.

The following foods typically contain *higher* levels of histamine.

- Fermented dairy products, such as cheese (especially aged), yogurt, sour cream, and buttermilk
- Fermented vegetables, such as sauerkraut and kimchi
- Pickles or pickled veggies
- Kombucha
- Cured or fermented meats, such as sausages, salami, and fermented ham
- Wine, beer, alcohol, and champagne
- Fermented soy products, such as tempeh, miso, soy sauce, and natto
- Fermented grains, such as sourdough bread
- Tomatoes
- Eggplant
- Spinach
- Frozen, salted, or canned fish, such as sardines and tuna
- Vinegar
- Tomato ketchup and some mustard formulations

The foods in the following list may cause the *release* of histamine from our immune cells.

- Most citrus fruits (e.g., lemon, lime, oranges, and so on)
- Cocoa and chocolate
- Walnuts, peanuts
- Papaya, pineapples, plums, kiwifruit, and bananas
- Legumes
- Tomatoes
- Wheat germ
- Most vinegars
- Additives (e.g., benzoate, sulphites, nitrites, glutamate, and food dyes)

These foods are reported to block DAO enzyme:

- Alcohol
- Black tea
- Energy drinks
- Yerba maté tea

You may be overwhelmed by the lists above. I sure was the first time I looked at them.

CAUTION: Do Not Remove Too Many Food Groups from Your Child's Diet!

I'm going to be a bit of a broken record on this topic, but it is not safe to remove too many food groups from your child's diet, especially all at once! With histamine-sensitive kids, we have to be careful that they do not become malnourished. I like to think of it as a replacement diet rather than an elimination diet; any food removed needs to be replaced with a histamine-friendly substitute.

When we are trying to heal our kids from something like eczema, we tend to grasp onto the things that we can control. Food is one of those things, and so we think that's the only thing that will help them. But we have to remember that food is just one part of an overall approach to healing.

Please keep in mind that each person is an individual, and not every high-histamine food will bother everyone. It is good to change up what you are eating and not eat the exact same things each day.

Histamine-Rich Foods: Eat This Instead!

In working to heal leaky gut, food elimination can be daunting. Instead of focusing on all the things we can't have in regard to histamines, we are going to approach it from an "eat this instead" point of view. There are a number of foods I would simply avoid because of the amount of histamine. Foods with moderate histamine I would limit to once per day. We also cover some substitution options below.

High Histamine Foods to Avoid or Limit

AVOID	LIMIT
artificial colors	avocados
artificial flavors	bananas
preservatives	peaches
chocolate, cocoa powder	pineapple
strawberries	spinach
kombucha	tomato
dairy	fermented foods like sauerkraut
spinach	leftovers
soy sauce	citrus
tofu/tempeh	mushrooms
processed vegan meat	dried fruit
bacon	
pepperoni, cured meats	
sausage	
hot dogs	
raw egg whites	
canned fish	
smoked salmon	
inflammatory oils, like vegetable and canola	

Figure 8.1

High Histamine Food Substitutions

Foods	Substitutes
Banana	Applesauce or pumpkin in baking
Spinach	Kale
Strawberries	Blueberries or cherries
Leftovers from dinner	Freeze them immediately and use later
Marinara-based pasta sauces	Garlic, olive oil, and leafy herbs
Dairy	Coconut milk, hemp milk, nut milk if tolerated
Soy sauce	Bragg Coconut Liquid Aminos
Eggplant	Summer squash
Walnuts, cashews, and peanuts	Pistachios or almonds
Candy	Juice Plus gummies
French fries	Homemade sweet potato fries
Dairy or soy	Violife cheeses or coconut yogurt
Hot dogs	Grass-fed beef burgers
Regular ketchup	Carrot ketchup (Noble Made has one, and there are recipes you can find online to make it at home)

Figure 8.2

Environment Can Also Play a Role in Histamine Production and Release

Pollen and dust mites can bring in extra histamine, so checking your air quality is a must! Here are some tips.

1. Use an air filter. (I love the Air Doctor.)
2. Change your heat/AC filters routinely.
3. Vacuum often.
4. Brush your pet outside.
5. Leave your shoes at the door.
6. Change your pillows (avoid feather/down pillows, and use dust covers).
7. Wash anything fluffy, like blankets and stuffed animals, every week.
8. Cover mattresses in allergen protectors.
9. Check for mold in your home.

Improve DAO Enzyme Activity

There are several micronutrients that help improve DAO activity. Most of these are found in our diet, so a supplement is not necessarily needed, but this highlights the importance of maintaining micronutrient levels in our body.

- Vitamin D
- Zinc
- Copper
- Iron
- Vitamin B6
- Magnesium
- Methylated B12

Last, the gut microbiome needs TLC to reduce histamine. (See Chapter 4 for more information on gut health.) Gut infection and overgrowth of certain gram-negative bacteria, such as *E. coli* and *Salmonella typhimurium*, can lead to increased histamine release.[76, 77] In our guts, we have many varieties of bacteria, but if there are more bad guys than good guys (a situation known as dysbiosis), things like histamines can become an issue. Why does this happen? These four factors are major contributors:

1. Medications (antibiotics, antacids, and NSAIDS)
2. Stress
3. Poor diet choices
4. Illness

By now, you might be tempted to reach for a probiotic to restore balance. But proceed with caution because some strains of probiotics can increase histamine levels. The following

---

76 https://pubmed.ncbi.nlm.nih.gov/16259743/
77 https://pubmed.ncbi.nlm.nih.gov/18606698/

strains produce histamines and are found in most yogurts and fermented foods:

- *Lactobacillus casei*
- *Lactobacillus reuteri*
- *Lactobacillus bulgaricus*
- *Streptococcus thermophilus*
- *Lactobacillus delbrueckii*
- *Lactobacillus helveticus*

If all the information on histamines is overwhelming to you, then you should feel right at home. It was foreign to me as well. Histamines were not my first consideration when I met Oliver, and I had never made a diagnosis of histamine intolerance. This is not something I learned about in medical school many years ago. For this very reason, I created a systematic approach in my online Eczema Transformation Program to address histamines with food substitutions, recipes, and supplement protocols. (I recommend that families who are battling a histamine issue get help from a professional who understands the fine details of histamine physiology.)

As I went through Oliver's story, a picture began to emerge in my mind. This was a child whose immune system was overeager to fight anything.

When I mentioned to the residents-in-training my suspicion that histamine intolerance was the underlying issue in Oliver's case, they looked at me like I was crazy. I explained my rationale, and we decided to proceed with a food sensitivity test. When Oliver's test results arrived, we couldn't believe our eyes. He was reacting to every single food on the list. Histamine intolerance was the only thing that would explain these startling results.

I formulated a plan to place Oliver on a low-histamine diet, and instituted some of the additional measures mentioned above to reduce his histamine load. When we saw him again in a month, his mom was smiling—always a telltale sign. She said that within two to three weeks, Oliver's eczema had begun to improve, and so did his appetite. I asked Oliver how he was feeling and he responded, "My belly doesn't hurt anymore!" I was so relieved. This was a new diagnosis for me, and I had gone with my gut.

Of note, we had also started Oliver on several micronutrients, including vitamin D, given the high prevalence of vitamin D deficiency and the fact that vitamin D is important for DAO function. Vitamin D, as well as a number of other micronutrients, can play an important role in the modulation of our immune system and in the management of eczema. In the next chapter, we will go through the micronutrients I feel are most influential in the eczema process.

Chapter Takeaways

- Histamines are an important part of our normal immune system. They play an integral role in acute allergic reactions and protect us from dangerous toxins.
- Elevated histamine levels that are due to diet, leaky gut, stress, environment, nutritional deficiencies, drugs, hormones, and DAO enzyme deficiency lead to chronic inflammation and disease, such as eczema.
- I recommend reducing histamine levels via substitution diets, environmental cleanup, and improving DAO function. Intermittent use of antihistamines can be helpful for flares and, in severe cases, long-term use might be necessary until gut healing is achieved or complete.

Additional resources to help you reduce environmental allergens in your home can be found on our book resources page by scanning the QR code below.

9

Decoding the Micronutrient-Eczema Connection

There are a number of diseases that are clearly caused by a vitamin or mineral deficiency, though we tend to believe these problems have been eradicated in the modern world. For example, vitamin C deficiency, which historically affected sailors after long periods at sea, leads to scurvy, a disease characterized by bleeding gums, bruising, and fatigue. Rickets, caused by a vitamin D deficiency, leads to weak bones, with bowed legs, recurrent fractures, and stunted growth. Iodine deficiency results in goiter, hypothyroidism, and developmental delays because of iodine's importance in thyroid function.

The diseases above only occur in cases of severe malnutrition, and we tend to dismiss these concerns in developed countries such as the United States. But I am here to tell you that disease resulting from micronutrient deficiency remains a major problem worldwide, even in developed countries. What really gets missed are the problems that develop from milder, partial deficiencies.

Recognizing these more moderate states of deficiency was a major breakthrough for me in my management of eczema. A memorable patient experience opened my eyes to the world of micronutrient deficiencies.

Hope for Better Skin

Nine-month-old Hope was brought in by her mother, Dianne, for persistent skin inflammation and rash, which I determined was eczema. She was covered in eczema from head to toe, with some areas (such as her belly and face) much worse than others. After examining Hope, I began my explanation of the pathophysiology of eczema and its origins and laid out my plan for treatment. Hope's family ate quite a bit of processed foods and sugar, so this was one of my first areas of attack. So far, the family was on board. I discussed adding fresh fruits and vegetables, whole organic foods, and correcting some probable micronutrient deficiencies with diet.

I then added that if Hope was not eating adequate amounts of food to correct nutritional deficiencies, we may need to add some supplements to her diet. Dianne initially fell silent, then looked up with concern. "We are really struggling financially, and I don't think we can afford to buy supplements. In fact, we have saved every extra penny just to make this appointment." She was totally distraught. Upon further discussion, we decided to proceed with my normal gut-healing protocol by addressing diet, environment, and stress but limiting the use of supplements owing to their financial constraints.

Given Hope's history, I did feel vitamin D and probiotics were important for her healing process, and her parents agreed to try just those two. I saw Hope again about a month later to check her progress, and asked Dianne how things were going. She said,

"I really haven't noticed much of a difference yet, but it's taken us a little while to get the dietary changes down." I wasn't concerned, as many patients don't see changes in the first month. We scheduled Hope for another appointment in about two months, which would have been three months from the start of treatment.

Hope arrived at her 3-month follow-up appointment, and I knew things weren't good the moment I saw Dianne. She was nearly in tears. "We have been doing everything you said. The diet, changing home products, wet wraps, stress reduction, but she just doesn't seem to be getting any better. I am really frustrated."

So was I. I believed they had been reliably sticking to the program. I was hesitant to add anything because of how cost-conscious they were. But I knew I needed to change something. I remembered Albert Einstein's quote, "Insanity is doing the same thing over and over and expecting different results."

One part of the program I had changed for Hope's care was limiting vitamin and mineral supplementation because of cost. With that in mind, I convinced Dianne to add a zinc supplement because many children are zinc deficient and lack of zinc has been linked to eczema (and it's also relatively inexpensive). They left the office that day with zinc in hand and plans to return in one month.

When they returned the following month, I entered the exam room with trepidation. Dianne's face relayed no clue as to how things were going. She held Hope facing her, so I couldn't see if Hope's face had cleared of any eczema. As I began to ask about the last month, Dianne blurted out, "You're not going to believe this. It's so much better than it has ever been. I can't believe that just adding zinc made such a huge difference."

Hope's family sticks out in my mind (we'll return to her story at the end of this chapter) because they were really struggling financially and I had to adjust a number of my recommendations because of cost, particularly involving supplements. Ironically, the problem I usually encounter is that a family wants to solve a child's eczema with supplements alone. One of the most common questions I get regarding eczema is, "What vitamins or supplements should I use for my child's eczema?" As I have been explaining throughout this book, eczema cannot be treated by a pill alone. Yet Americans, with their pill-hungry attitude, want to punch the big red "Easy" button to solve the problem, rather than do the hard work of cleaning up their lives.

The Malnourished Obese

As we begin to discuss the role of micronutrients in eczema development, I think we need to take a step back to look more closely at the implications of the Western diet. Around the world, countries that have adopted the Western diet have also struggled with staggering rates of obesity and autoimmune diseases such as eczema. The ironic twist is that most of the people suffering from obesity are also malnourished. It seems like an oxymoron to refer to the obese as malnourished, but the facts speak for themselves. One sobering example is a German study showing that 96 percent of overweight and obese children were vitamin D deficient.[78] Further studies have revealed that being deficient in vitamin D is, in and of itself, a risk factor for obesity.[79]

My goal here is not to rant about the obesity epidemic; it's to reframe the way you look at nutrition. Rather than focusing on the quantity of our calories, we need to focus on the quality

---

78 https://www.ncbi.nlm.nih.gov/pmc/articles/PMC6406072/

79 https://pubmed.ncbi.nlm.nih.gov/23924693/#:~:text=Low%20 25(OH)D%20levels%20correlated%20with%20high%20 body%20fat,leading%20to%20diabetes%20type%202.

of those calories. One calorie of a micronutrient-rich food, like kale, is very different than one calorie of Goldfish crackers (my children's favorite, at one point.) The high-calorie, low-micronutrient Western diet has led to a malnourishment epidemic—an obese population lacking essential vitamins and minerals.

How did this happen? Technology has allowed food companies to scale production exponentially, but this has come at the cost of quality. The commercialization of crop production with extensive use of pesticides, herbicides, synthetic fertilizers, lack of crop rotation, and genetically modified organisms (GMOs) has changed our food and depleted the soil. Remember, the minerals we obtain through our foods are sourced through the soil during growth of the plant. Additionally, large-scale farms have also changed the way they feed livestock and poultry, often feeding the animals with micronutrient-poor feed. As a result, every bite we put in our mouths likely contains fewer micronutrients than it did many years ago.

The Eczema Connection

Hopefully by now I have convinced you that eczema is not the result of one thing. It's a truly multifactorial disease. Micronutrient deficiencies are just other pieces of the puzzle that need to be addressed when tackling eczema. Although there are likely dozens of vitamin and mineral deficiencies that will ultimately be found to play a role in eczema, I have found three to be the most common: vitamin D, zinc, and omega-3s. I want to discuss each of these at length, as I think it will lead to a better understanding of the dietary implications of eczema.

I also want to emphasize that the best way to correct micronutrient deficiencies is by eating whole foods rich in those molecules. But as stated previously, the reality is that 6–10 percent of

Americans live in a food desert. And that number jumps to 20 percent in rural areas.[80] In many of those communities, the only way to obtain adequate amounts of these vital nutrients may be to supplement them. This opens up a whole other can of worms, given that the supplement industry is like the wild west, with little government oversight, many poor-quality products, and some predatory manufacturers. With all that in mind, let's look at the big three essentials for combating eczema.

Vitamin D

Vitamin D (aka calciferol) is actually NOT present in many foods. If you read a label that says "great source of vitamin D," it's because the manufacturer has added it to the food. Humans generally derive over 90 percent of our vitamin D from that great big ball of burning gas in the sky—our sun. Our skin is pretty darn smart and uses the UV rays from the sun to synthesize vitamin D.

However, humans are spending less and less time in the sun. In fact, vitamin D deficiency is a growing global problem, especially in kids. Numerous studies indicate that up to 60 percent of children have low levels of vitamin D.[81, 82, 83] Figure 9.1 shows the recommended daily intake of vitamin D based on age.

80 https://www.usda.gov/media/blog/2011/05/03/interactive-web-tool-maps-food-deserts-provides-key-data

81 https://www.ncbi.nlm.nih.gov/pmc/articles/PMC5073161/

82 https://pubmed.ncbi.nlm.nih.gov/18524739/

83 https://academic.oup.com/jpubhealth/article/40/4/721/4953712

Recommended Daily Intake of Vitamin D

Age Group	Recommended Dietary Allowance (RDA) per day	Tolerable Upper Intake Level (UL) per day
Infants 0–6 months	400 IU (10 mcg)*	1000 IU (25 mcg)
Infants 7–12 months	400 IU (10 mcg)*	1500 IU (38 mcg)
Children 1–3 years	600 IU (15 mcg)	2500 IU (63 mcg)
Children 4–8 years	600 IU (15 mcg)	3000 IU (75 mcg)
Children and Adults 9–70 years	600 IU (15 mcg)	4000 IU (100 mcg)
Adults > 70 years	800 IU (20 mcg)	4000 IU (100 mcg)
Pregnancy & Lactation	600 IU (15 mcg)	4000 IU (100 mcg)

* Adequate Intake rather than Recommended Dietary Allowance

Figure 9.1

Babies are particularly vulnerable, as they must get all of their vitamin D from the mother's breast milk (or formula) because they are rarely in the sun. Unfortunately, between 18 and 84 percent of mothers worldwide are also vitamin D deficient, depending on where they live.[84]

Additional studies suggest that children born to mothers with low vitamin D *intake* (regardless of serum vitamin D level) during pregnancy have an increased prevalence of eczema.[85] Supporting the vitamin D theory are studies showing that children born during autumn and winter have a higher prevalence of eczema compared to children born in spring and summer.[86] And the farther north (or south) you live from the equator correlates with an increasing risk of eczema development—another reason we should all live on a beautiful sunny beach in the tropics!

---

84 https://www.ncbi.nlm.nih.gov/pmc/articles/PMC5064090/

85 https://pubmed.ncbi.nlm.nih.gov/19840962/

86 https://pubmed.ncbi.nlm.nih.gov/17346293/

Here Comes the Sun

Adding to the importance of sunshine, one study showed that eczema sufferers from Norway (63rd parallel north) who were sent to the Canary Islands (28th parallel north) had dramatic improvements in their eczema. Researchers felt this improvement was likely from vitamin D elevations.[87] Individuals with darker skin (i.e., Black, Hispanic, or Indian) are less able to synthesize vitamin D in their skin; thus, they are more commonly vitamin D deficient AND—you guessed it—they have much higher rates of eczema.

Additionally, an American study showed that eczema sufferers also had higher risk of fractures! Why? Vitamin D, of course, which most people recognize as being important for bones. As well, many kids with eczema also take steroids, which weaken bones!

Many more studies have shown an association between eczema development and low vitamin D levels, but they are beyond the scope of this chapter.[88, 89]

Why We Need D

In eczema, vitamin D directly suppresses skin inflammation by increasing the production of an important anti-inflammatory protein: Interleukin 10 (IL-10).[90] It plays an important role in the general regulation of our immune systems, and its absence can lead to autoimmune problems such as eczema. As we discussed in the histamine chapter, vitamin D appears to have a crucial role in stabilizing mast cells—the pinata-like cells that burst open with

---

[87] https://pubmed.ncbi.nlm.nih.gov/17073869/
[88] https://pubmed.ncbi.nlm.nih.gov/23751100/
[89] https://pubmed.ncbi.nlm.nih.gov/24383670/
[90] https://pubmed.ncbi.nlm.nih.gov/20194632/

major inflammatory consequences. Last, it increases antimicrobial activity against staph infections.

Fun fact: people afflicted with eczema tend to have higher levels of *Staphylococcus aureus* (aka *S. aureus*, or staph) on their skin. Vitamin D (via supplements or the sun) stimulates skin cells to produce a protein (cathelicidin) that fights against staph.

There are likely many more mechanisms involving vitamin D in our bodies that we don't yet understand. It seems pretty obvious to me that one of the first steps in treating eczema is to get vitamin D levels elevated—NOT starting high doses of steroid creams! Crushing the immune system with steroids and cancer-treating drugs is not the best way to approach eczema—but Big Pharma companies are making billions from those drugs.

In my online Eczema Transformation Program, I walk families through the supplement protocols and dosing, while troubleshooting any side effects that may be encountered. Moreover, during the weekly live calls, we discuss various supplements and remedies discovered on Google and I help families figure out whether those are worth trying.

How to Raise Vitamin D Levels

The first option is to get a bit of sunshine in your kids' lives, if possible. Many parents are terrified about sun exposure in their kids—fair enough. So, put some sunscreen on them and force them outside! It seems intuitive that sunscreen would block the formation of vitamin D, but studies have not shown a dramatic reduction in vitamin D production when sunscreen is used.[91] This may be because we seem to be terrible at applying it effectively, don't use it frequently enough, and don't use adequate

---

91 https://pubmed.ncbi.nlm.nih.gov/30945275/

sun protection factor (SPF). Studies have shown that as little as 5 minutes daily in the sun, preferably between 10:00 a.m. and 4:00 p.m., can significantly raise vitamin D levels—and kids should be outside more, anyway![92]

Next, maximize food sources of vitamin D when possible. Figure 9.2 shows foods high in vitamin D.

Foods High in Vitamin D

Food	IUs per serving	Percent of RDA
Cod liver oil (1 tablespoon)	1,360	340
Swordfish (cooked, 3 ounces)	566	142
Sockeye salmon (cooked, 3 ounces)	447	112
Tuna fish (canned in water, drained, 3 ounces)	154	39
Sardines (canned in oil, drained, 2 sardines)	46	12
Beef liver (cooked, 3 ounces)	42	11
Egg (1 large, vitamin D is found in yolk)	41	10
Ready-to-eat cereal (fortified, 3/4-1 cup)	40	10

Figure 9.2

Assuming your kids are like mine, they probably aren't going to crack open some cod liver oil for breakfast or snack on a can of sardines after school. But let me tell you who eats sardines well: babies. I recommend sardines as one of the first foods for babies, even if the parents find them gross. Anywhere you can add these products into your cooking will help. Also, for the rare times you do have processed foods, choose ones fortified with vitamin D.

---

[92] https://ods.od.nih.gov/factsheets/VitaminD-HealthProfessional/#en13

After maximizing sun and food, supplementation may be required to bring those vitamin D levels back up. Families who live in northern climates during the winter months may have limited access to sunshine and may find supplementation necessary. It's rare that I recommend one supplement to everyone, but that exception is typically vitamin D because vitamin D deficiency is a global epidemic.[93]

If you Google vitamin D, you will be inundated with products and suggestions. So, how the heck do you choose? Before we take a nerdy yet thrilling ride into the world of vitamin D supplementation, I want to make a few comments about supplements in general.

A Word of Caution on Supplements

I strongly urge families to get their micronutrients via fresh fruits and vegetables, whole foods, organic meats, and wild-caught fish, as discussed in the previous chapters. If you do take supplements, beware—there is very little oversight out there in supplement land. I tell my patients to be wary of supplements sold on Amazon or similar sites. One study showed that the actual amount of micronutrients contained in randomly selected supplements ranged from 9 percent to 146 percent of what the label actually stated.[94]

In the United States, you can look for labels that include the Current Good Manufacturing Practices (CGMP) logo, as these products have met a minimal standard to avoid gross contamination. Despite CGMP oversight, a 2010 U.S. Government Accountability Office report revealed that an analysis of forty dietary

[93] https://www.ncbi.nlm.nih.gov/pmc/articles/PMC5394390/

[94] https://pubmed.ncbi.nlm.nih.gov/23400578/

supplements found trace amounts of one or more of lead, arsenic, mercury, cadmium, or pesticides in 93 percent of samples.[95]

For true confidence in supplement composition, you want approval from a third-party testing company. Two major *nonprofit* companies in the United States are the National Sanitation Foundation (NSF) and U.S. Pharmacopeia (USP), which both provide accurate and reliable supplement testing.

Reliable third-party testing is mandatory for supplements.

Two newer *for-profit* testers have also emerged: ConsumerLab.com and UL. Pretty much all the other "verified by" or "approved" stamps on bottles are meaningless. For this type of testing, I tend to trust the nonprofit companies to give me unbiased data. The bottom line: reliable third-party testing is mandatory for supplements.

These are the labels to look for to verify CGMP, and are the best-known third-party testers.

[95] US Government Accountability Office. Herbal Dietary Supplements: Examples of Deceptive or Questionable Marketing Practices and Potentially Dangerous Advice. Washington, DC: US Government Accountability Office; 2010. pp. 10–662T.

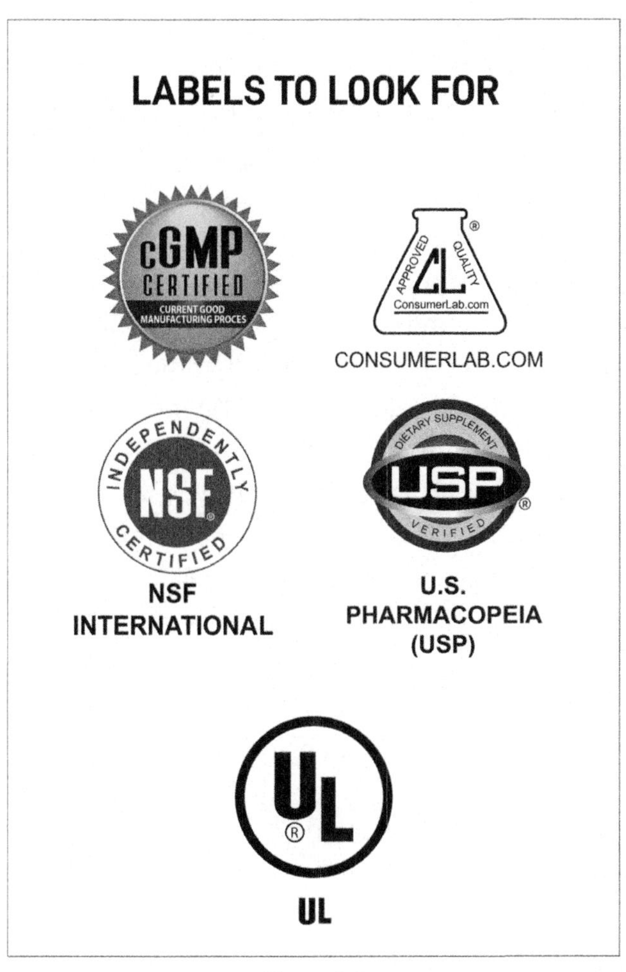

Figure 9.3

Understanding Vitamin D Supplements

There are two primary types of vitamin D: D2 (aka ergocalciferol) and D3 (aka cholecalciferol). Both forms of vitamin D are readily available as supplements, and both have been shown to be effective. Typically, D3 comes from animals (it's also the type that our skin makes), while D2 typically comes from plants.

This means that if you are a strict vegan, you may want to choose a D2 source (although one company now has made D3 from lichen). Debate exists around which form is better at raising vitamin D levels, but recent studies suggest that D3 has the edge and is a bit more effective.[96]

Now, we need to dive into the weeds of physiology a bit to discuss additional aspects of vitamin D supplementation.

To understand some of the minutiae of vitamin D, we need to review how vitamin D is absorbed and its mechanism of action. If ingested, vitamin D (either D2 or D3) moves into the small intestine, where it must mix with bile salts. Because vitamin D is a fat-soluble vitamin, it needs to mix with fat to be absorbed. The bile salts surround the vitamin D in a layer of fat and allow absorption. Bile salts are stored in the gallbladder. People who have had their gallbladders removed are at risk for vitamin D deficiency. This is why many vitamin D supplements also provide a fat/lipid/oil source within them. The vitamin D is turned into its active form in the kidney and begins to exert its effects around the body.

Once we have decided whether we'll take D3 or D2, we must also choose a form: liquid, spray, pill, or powder. It's overwhelming. Lots of studies on this exist as well, but many of them are sponsored by the supplement manufacturer, so you need to take them with a grain of salt.

As we discussed, vitamin D needs to be wrapped in fat to be absorbed in our gut. Science has created ways to wrap the vitamin D molecules inside fat before it even gets to our bellies. Packing the vitamin D in a liposome—a process called microencapsulation—allows larger amounts of the vitamin to be carried and provides delivery all the way to the tissues.

---

[96] https://www.ncbi.nlm.nih.gov/pmc/articles/PMC4971338/

Studies have shown that supplemental nutrients, such as vitamin C, vitamin D, and glutathione, are more effectively absorbed when carried in liposomes.[97] Although more study is needed, it looks like liposomal vitamin D3 may have the highest absorption rate.

What about capsules and powders? Your body treats these two formulations the same. Once the powder is ingested and moves to the small intestine, the bile salts from the gallbladder wrap the vitamin D in fat, which then gets absorbed in the intestines.

So, does higher absorption mean better results? Not necessarily.

There is no convincing data at this point that one form of vitamin D is clinically superior to any other. Some forms may raise vitamin D levels a bit faster, but that hasn't translated to significant reduction in eczema symptoms compared to other forms. I think focusing on a quality, third-party-tested product is the most important factor.

There is no convincing data at this point that one form of vitamin D is clinically superior to any other.

Why Does My Vitamin D Supplement Also Contain Vitamin K?

You will notice that many vitamin D supplements also contain K2—what the heck? Why would we need vitamin K? Here's the long-winded answer. You may remember that vitamin D is very important in the regulation of calcium in our bodies—but so is vitamin K.

---

97 https://www.ncbi.nlm.nih.gov/pmc/articles/PMC6631968/

It turns out that vitamins D and K work in close harmony to manage calcium regulation. Vitamin K may actually help protect us from the negative aspects of vitamin D. If we get too much vitamin D, it will cause our calcium levels to be too high (though this is rare). That excess calcium can get deposited on the walls of blood vessels, and calcification is responsible for much of our cardiovascular (CV) diseases.

Vitamin K takes that extra calcium and directs it toward bone and other useful places, to protect our CV system. Thus, by combining vitamin D and K, we gain CV benefits in addition to the bone and skin benefits.

So, why K1 versus K2?

I am really trying NOT to confuse you. There are two primary types of vitamin K: K1 and K2. K1 is found in green leafy vegetables and is the predominant form in the human diet. K2 is found in highly fermented foods, such as sauerkraut, natto (a Japanese food made of fermented soybeans), cheese, liver, and yogurt. It is also produced by bacteria in our guts (see Figure 9.4).

K1 and K2 actually have different functions in the body, and both are necessary. Since K2 is better absorbed in our guts, and less common in our diets, it is the one added to supplements.

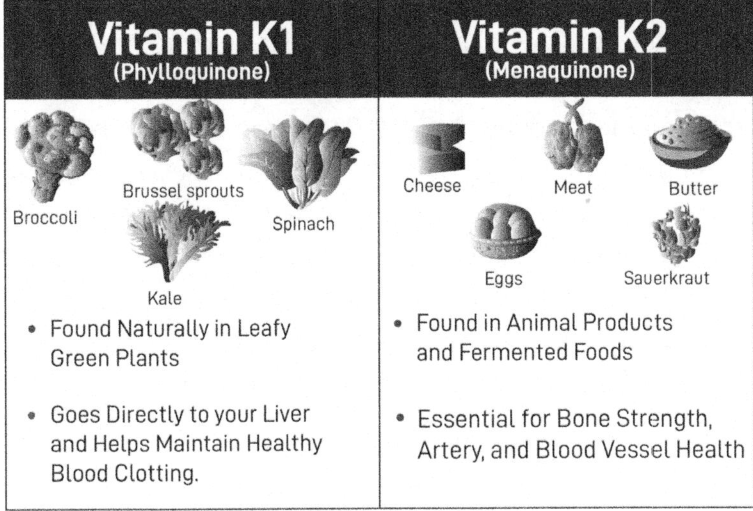

Figure 9.4

The Verdict on Vitamin D

Before I give you my verdict, I want to repeat something: GET YOUR KIDS OUTSIDE! I can't stress this enough. No supplement company on Earth has been shown to be better than the sun at cranking out high-quality vitamin D.

Now, with that off my chest, I will give you the bottom line. Current research shows that liposomal packaged vitamin D3 may have the highest absorption rate compared to other forms.[98] But, again, it has NOT been shown to be more effective at reducing symptoms of eczema (more studies are needed). There are even other factors to consider, like binders, alcohol, natural flavors, sugar, fillers, and excipients, which are all the "extra" ingredients in your supplements.

---

98 https://www.ncbi.nlm.nih.gov/pmc/articles/PMC6631968/

Basically, there is no perfect vitamin D supplement. I think getting vitamin D from a reputable source is probably the most important factor, given the high variability in contents and quality. My current favorite—and the one I use in my online Eczema Transformation Program—is NOT a liposomal form. The current liposomal forms are filled with added sugars, flavors, and fillers that I don't like. Currently, I use *DrAnaMaria-Approved Liquid D3 with K2* because it is super clean and without added ingredients. It is not NSF certified, but it is third-party tested by a reliable lab. You can check out other reliable third-party-tested supplements at my online store. https://shop.dranamaria.com

Zinc

Zinc is involved in thousands of vital processes within our body and has been used for decades to treat numerous skin conditions. While about half of the body's zinc is in the bones, nearly 6 percent of it is contained in the skin. Zinc also plays an important role in maintaining proper reproductive function, immune status, and wound repair. Last, it blocks the production of inflammatory proteins by our skin cells.

Zinc maintains the function of many of our white blood cells, which are central to the inflammatory processes seen with eczema. Mast cells are stabilized by zinc. Zinc also possesses antioxidant properties and has been found useful in preventing sun-induced skin damage and reducing the incidence of cancers.[99]

Less known is zinc's vital importance in growth—particularly in infants, teens during puberty, and pregnant women. Deficiencies can cause significant growth defects, in addition to skin abnormalities. For kids, zinc is key for normal growth. Maintaining

[99] https://www.ncbi.nlm.nih.gov/pmc/articles/PMC4120804/

proper levels of zinc can prevent significant growth retardation, loss of appetite, impaired immune function, hair loss, diarrhea, delayed sexual maturation, impotence, hypogonadism in males, eye and skin lesions, weight loss, delayed healing of wounds, taste abnormalities, and mental lethargy. (Wow, go zinc.)

When kids with eczema were studied, they were found to have lower levels of zinc in their blood and hair, compared to individuals without eczema.[100] Several randomized controlled trials have shown that kids receiving zinc supplementation had significant improvements in the extent and severity of their eczema, as well as reduced itching compared with the group not receiving supplementation.[101,102] Given this association and the high prevalence of zinc deficiency, I think it's important to ensure all patients with eczema are getting adequate levels of zinc in their diet or supplementing.

Not Enough Zinc

Zinc deficiency is a common problem. An estimated one-third of the world's population suffers from zinc deficiency (with very high prevalence in Southeast Asia, sub-Saharan Africa, and other developing countries).[103] Many foods once rich in zinc are no longer reliable sources because zinc levels have been depleted in the soils that grow the crops. The map in Figure 9.5 shows that much of the world has zinc-deficient soil.

---

[100] https://pubmed.ncbi.nlm.nih.gov/30801794/
[101] https://www.medicaljournals.se/acta/content/html/10.2340/00015555-1772
[102] https://pubmed.ncbi.nlm.nih.gov/31745908/
[103] https://www.ncbi.nlm.nih.gov/books/NBK493231/

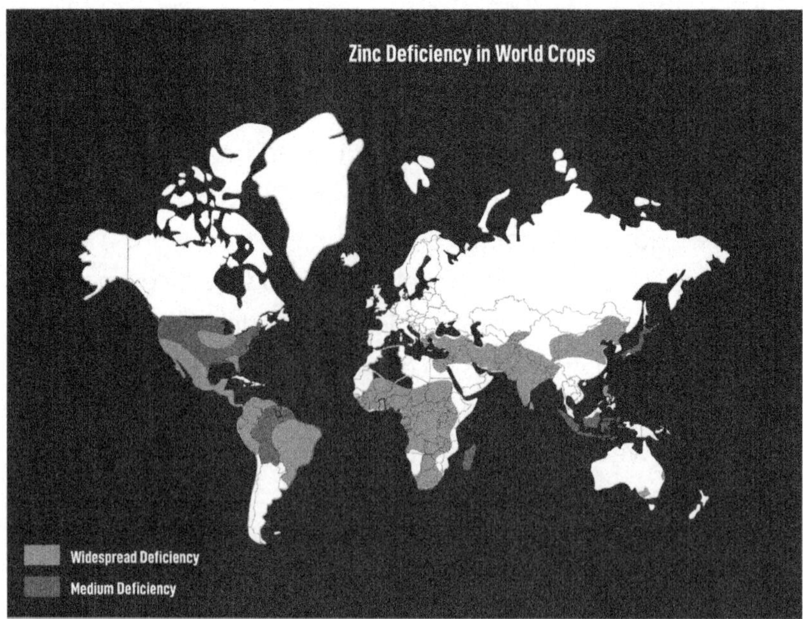

Figure 9.5

Given that our bodies have no zinc storage capability, we must get ours through daily consumption. Zinc is absorbed in the intestine and our bodies are efficient at increasing or decreasing the amount of zinc absorbed depending on need.[104]

In my practice, infants and other patients with highly selective diets are most at risk of zinc deficiency. Given that animal foods are the primary source of zinc, people following a vegan or other animal-free diet are at particular risk. The chart below shows foods that are high in zinc.

104 https://www.ncbi.nlm.nih.gov/pmc/articles/PMC4120804/#B5

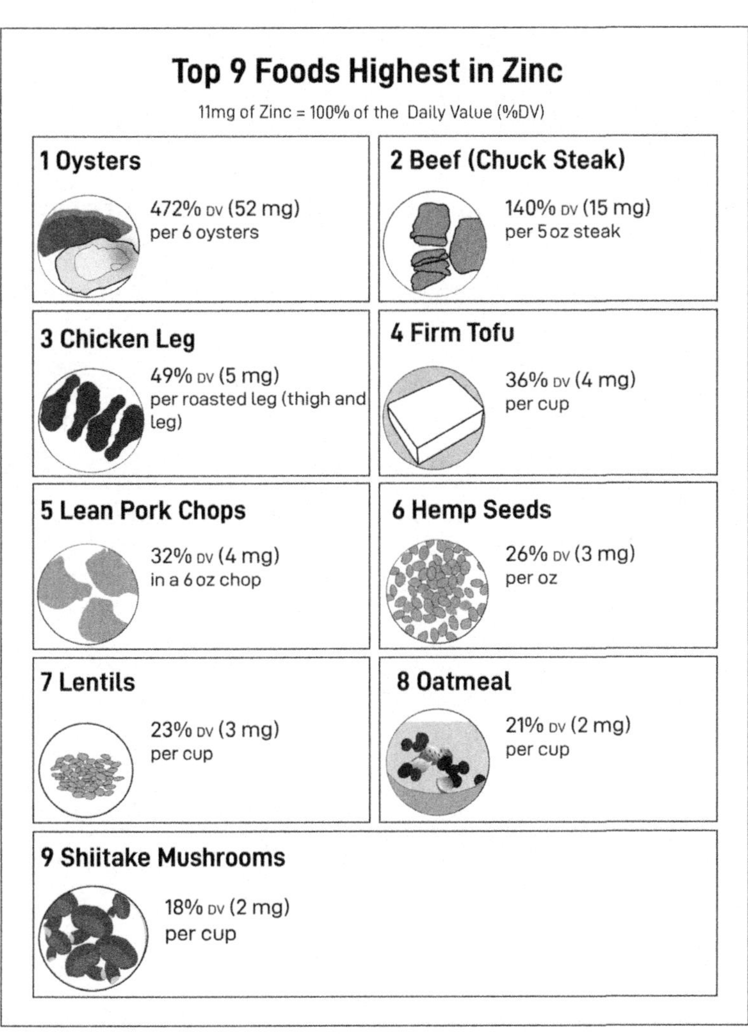

Figure 9.6

I can't speak for everyone, but when my kids were small, oysters were not high on their list of most desired foods in the old lunchbox. Animal foods like meat, eggs, fish, and oysters are rich in zinc. Most Americans get their zinc from meat and poultry.

Vegetarians can get zinc from beans, nuts, and grains—but there's a catch. Although cereals and legumes (beans) contain moderate amounts of zinc, only 20–40 percent of the ingested mineral is absorbed. Plant sources of zinc contain phytates (aka phytic acid), which are antioxidant compounds. Phytates bind zinc and other minerals and block their absorption. So, you must eat significantly more beans to get your share of zinc because of this binding issue. One option is to soak beans or nuts in water for several hours before cooking, as this helps to remove phytates.

Last, many processed foods (like breakfast cereals) are fortified with zinc, but since you, my reader, are NOT giving your kids these garbage cereals, we can't rely on that for a zinc source ... right?

How Much Zinc Do You need?

How Much Zinc Do You Need?

Life stage	RDA	UL
0–6 months	2 mg/day	4 mg/day
7–12 months	3 mg/day	5 mg/day
1–3 years	3 mg/day	7 mg/day
4–8 years	5 mg/day	12 mg/day
9–13 years	8 mg/day	23 mg/day
14–18 years (female)	9 mg/day	34 mg/day
14–18 years (male)	11 mg/day	34 mg/day
19+ (female)	8 mg/day	40 mg/day
19+ (male)	11 mg/day	40 mg/day
During pregnancy (14–18 years)	12 mg/day	34 mg/day
During pregnancy (19+)	11 mg/day	40 mg/day
During lactation (14–18 years)	13 mg/day	34 mg/day
During lactation (19+)	12 mg/day	40 mg/day
No RDA exists for infants from birth to six months, so the Adequate Intake (AI) is listed instead. The Institute of Medicine bases this off of the mean intake of zinc in babies exclusively fed human milk.		

Figure 9.7

If your daily intake of zinc is low, or you are suffering from eczema, I would recommend zinc supplementation. Given some of the absorption issues discussed above, zinc needs to be attached to another substance. Often, it is *chelated* (combined to form complexes) with organic and amino acids, to increase its bioavailability or to ease absorption into the body. Although studies have shown that chelated zincs have higher levels of absorption than non-chelated forms, they have not been definitively shown to be better at reducing eczema symptoms.[105]

Also, some authors claim that one form of zinc is better against certain diseases than other forms (for example, some say that zinc acetate is better for colds). I question these claims and don't feel that one chelated form is better than any other. Some common forms of zinc include:

Chelated zincs

- Zinc gluconate
- Zinc acetate
- Zinc picolinate
- Zinc orotate
- Zinc citrate

Non-chelated or inorganic zincs

- Zinc sulfate
- Zinc oxide

In my online Eczema Transformation Program, I use *DrAna-Maria-Approved Zinc Gummies* or *Capsules*. They contain a chelated zinc that gives them better absorption. I also use a zinc gluconate liquid, as it is easy to take for kids of all ages and has a tolerable taste. Last, I advise families NOT to dose above the amounts recommended in the program, because zinc toxicity, though rare, can occur. Additionally, too much zinc can cause a copper

105 https://www.ncbi.nlm.nih.gov/pmc/articles/PMC3901420/

deficiency because the surplus of zinc competes with copper for absorption.

Omega-3 Fatty Acids

At some point, you may have been told that you should eat more fish or add fish oils to your diet to increase omega-3 intake. Omega-3s are unsaturated fatty acids that are an essential part of our diet. We cannot produce them, and they are vital to a number of processes in our body. There are three main types: one is derived from plants and the other two from fish.

Types of omega-3s

ALA

Alpha-linolenic acid (ALA) is a plant form of omega-3. It's found in flaxseed, chia seeds, walnuts, and canola and soybean oils. (I don't recommend canola or soybean oils.) ALA is an essential fatty acid (EFA) because our bodies can't make it and it can only be obtained from our diet. Figure 9.8 shows typical ALA levels in our food.

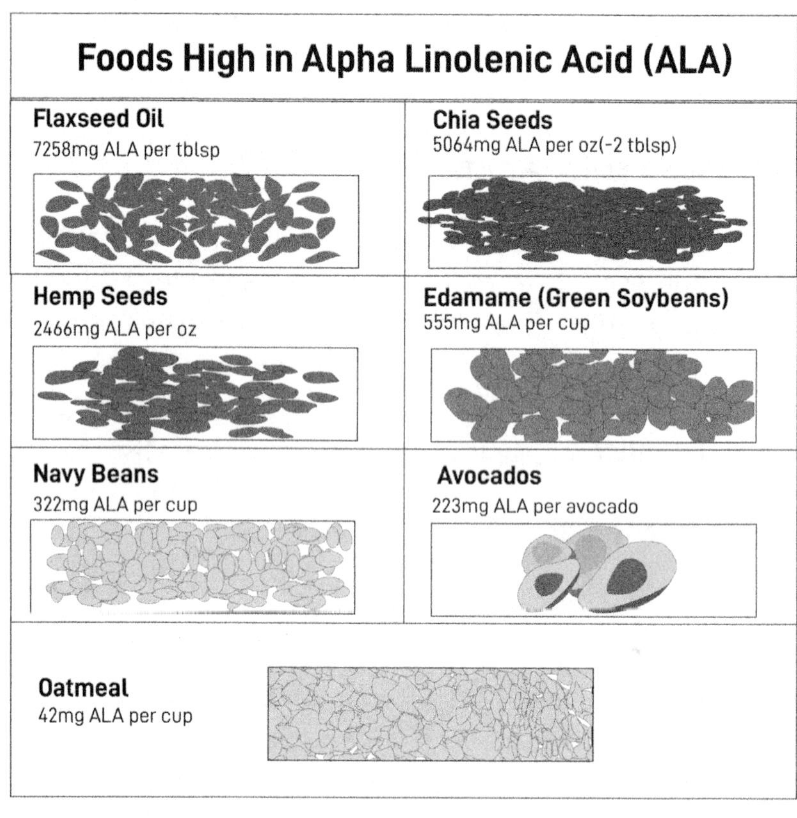

Figure 9.8

EPA and DHA

Eicosapentaenoic acid (EPA) and docosahexaenoic acid (DHA) are the marine forms of omega-3s. They are commonly found in cold-water fatty fish like salmon, herring, sardines, and mackerel. These fatty acids can be made from ALA in the body—but the conversion rate is poor, so we must get most of them from our diet. These two polyunsaturated fatty acids (PUFAs) found in fish (EPA and DHA) have been found to be the most beneficial because of their anti-inflammatory properties. Figure 9.9 shows average amounts of EPA and DHA in marine food sources.

Selected Food Sources of DHA and EPA

FOOD	GRAMS PER SERVING	
	DHA	EPA
Salmon, Atlantic, farmed, cooked, 3 oz	1.24.g	0.59.g
Salmon, Atlantic, wild, cooked, 3 oz	1.22.g	0.35.g
Herring, Atlantic, cooked, 3 oz	1.94.g	0.77.g
Sardines, canned in tomato sauce, drained, 3 oz	0.74.g	0.45.g
Mackerel, Atlantic, cooked, 3 oz	0.59.g	0.43.g
Salmon, pink, canned, drained, 3 oz	0.63.g	0.28.g
Trout, rainbow, wild, cooked, 3 oz	0.44.g	0.30.g
Oysters, eastern, wild, cooked, 3 oz	0.23.g	0.40.g
Sea bass, cooked, 3 oz	0.47.g	0.18.g
Shrimp, cooked, 3 oz	0.12.g	0.12.g
Lobster, cooked, 3 oz	0.07.g	0.10.g
Tuna, light, canned in water, drained, 3 oz	0.17.g	0.02.g
Scallops, cooked, 3 oz	0.09.g	0.06.g
Cod, Pacific, cooked, 3 oz	0.10.g	0.04.g
Tuna, yellowfin, cooked, 3 oz	0.09.g	0.01.g

Figure 9.9

Omega-3 functions

Omega-3s function to regulate the immune system by controlling cells that cause inflammation and producing proteins that slow the inflammatory process. In the skin, omega-3s have been found to improve barrier function, inhibit inflammation (particularly from UV light), and promote skin healing.[106] The body incorporates dietary fatty acids into cell membranes. When a cell membrane is healthy, the cell can hold water. In the skin, this results in cells being hydrated and soft. Figure 9.10 is an image of a skin cell with a lipid bilayer. The lipid bilayer is where omega-3 fatty acids congregate.

SKIN CELL WITH LIPID BILAYER

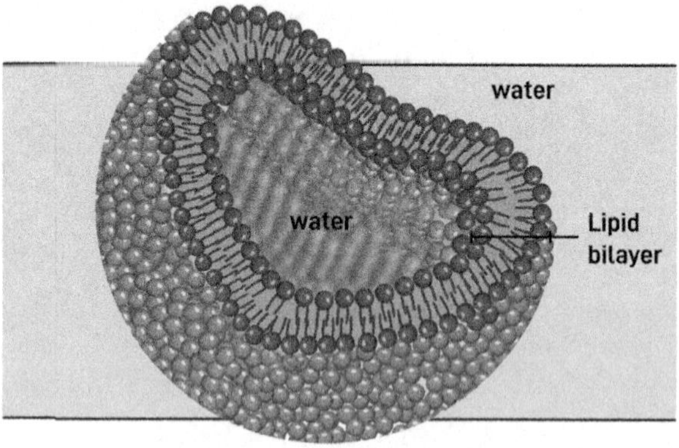

Figure 9.10

Eczema reduction

A number of studies have shown that using omega-3 supplements can reduce eczema symptoms, particularly itch-related scratching. However, the results have been inconsistent.[107,108] In a study of 3,285 Swedish children, researchers found that regular fish consumption

---

106 https://www.ncbi.nlm.nih.gov/pmc/articles/PMC6117694/

107 https://pubmed.ncbi.nlm.nih.gov/26882378/

108 https://www.ncbi.nlm.nih.gov/pubmed/26195090/

early in life may reduce the risk of allergies (particularly rhinitis and eczema) up to the age of twelve.[109] Animal studies have shown a clear benefit to the intake of oily fish or omega-3 supplements for skin inflammation, but human studies are lacking.[110] Studies not focused on the skin clearly show that omega-3 supplements reduce inflammation in the body and have cardiovascular benefits.[111] Thus, omega-3s are a mainstay of treatment for my eczema patients.

As an added benefit, omega-3s may help with brain processes in people with attention-deficit hyperactivity disorder (ADHD). In a 2018 review, international experts advised that omega-3 supplements may produce small but significant reductions in ADHD symptoms, while having a tolerable safety profile.[112] Omega-3s may minimize wound infections and speed up healing, which is useful in cases of discoloration caused by skin trauma. Also, evidence exists that fish oil may be beneficial in the treatment of acne, which can also cause long-term skin trauma.[113]

And for Mom, omega-3s help reduce the production of inflammatory compounds that contribute to the aging process.[114] (And we are all fighting the aging process!)

Too much omega-6

The benefits of omega-3s are in contrast to omega-6, which is another essential fatty acid found in vegetable oils, nuts, and seeds. Although omega-6 has benefits in the body, it can actually *turn on* inflammation. Arachidonic acid (AA), an omega-6, can increase immunoglobulin E (IgE) antibodies, which are central to allergic reactions and sensitivities. Omega-3 may displace the

---

[109] https://pubmed.ncbi.nlm.nih.gov/23576046/
[110] https://www.ncbi.nlm.nih.gov/pubmed/26195090/
[111] https://pubmed.ncbi.nlm.nih.gov/28900017/
[112] https://www.ncbi.nlm.nih.gov/pmc/articles/PMC6291899/
[113] https://pubmed.ncbi.nlm.nih.gov/24553997/
[114] https://www.ncbi.nlm.nih.gov/pmc/articles/PMC3575932/

AA and reduce the inflammatory proteins, therefore reducing the risk of allergic reactions.[115]

Omega-6 is meant to work in close harmony with omega-3 in regulating inflammation. Early humans typically ate a ratio of 1:1 omega-6 to omega-3. Our Western diet has now ballooned that ratio to almost 30:1, with omega-6 composing a large portion of our diet. This is largely due to the fact that vegetable oil, canola oil, corn oil, sunflower oil, safflower oil, and the like are put in a majority of our processed foods (think packaged snacks). This abnormal ratio may play a major role in the pro-inflammatory state of most Americans.

Figure 9.11 shows just how lopsided these ratios have become in many common cooking oils.

Cooking Oils and Omega Ratios

Cooking Oils	Omega-6: Omega-3 Ratio
Safflower oil	133:1
Sunflower oil	40:1
Corn oil	83:1
High-oleic sunflower oil	40:1
Sesame oil	42:1
Cottonseed oil	54:1
Grapeseed oil	676:1
Walnut oil	5:1
Hemp seed oil	3:1
Canola oil (expeller pressed)	2:1
High quality (low acidity) extra virgin olive oil	9:1
Flaxseed oil	1:4

Figure 9.11

[115] https://www.ncbi.nlm.nih.gov/pmc/articles/PMC4783952/

Omega-3 Supplement Options

In choosing an omega-3 supplement, there are several options but, in general, we want to get lots of the DHA and EPA variety of omega-3. Fish oil, made from the flesh of fatty fish such as salmon or mackerel, is the most common supplemental form of omega-3s. It contains EPA and DHA and comes in liquid or gel capsules.

Another specific type of fish oil is cod liver oil. It is made from the livers of cod, which is not a fatty fish. One benefit of cod liver oil is that it also contains vitamins A, D, and E—all of which are beneficial to eczema.

In my online Eczema Transformation Program there are a lot of kids allergic to fish. For those families, there are other options for omega-3: algal or flaxseed. The algal form is made from the same algae fish eat, providing them with the high levels of DHA and EPA that are in fish oils. The amount of DHA and EPA in the algal-sourced or flaxseed omegas is a bit lower, so getting the desired dose may involve taking additional capsules. Don't forget that dried seaweed snacks are a great source of plant-based omegas, as is flaxseed oil.

The Bottom Line for Hope

Given the large role that vitamin D, zinc, and omega-3s may play in the development of eczema, my treatment standard is to start new eczema patients on a supplement regimen of all three. These supplements are extremely safe, and given how common these deficiencies are, I think it's better to simply replace them rather than draw blood levels and determine the patients' level of deficiency.

I want to circle back to Hope, the eczema patient from the beginning of this chapter. As you may recall, Hope's mother, Dianne, wanted to avoid all supplements because of cost, so we did not start my typical supplement replacement of vitamin D, zinc, and omega-3s. Given our mounting frustration and Hope's failure to improve with dietary and environmental changes, I convinced Dianne to start zinc supplementation. When she returned to the office four weeks later, she couldn't believe the dramatic change. "Within a week or ten days, her skin began to change," Dianne explained. "At first I didn't believe it, but then it just kept getting better. I don't cringe anymore when I take her clothes off for bath time."

It was emotional for both of us. I know how hard it is to watch your child suffer. But what Dianne didn't appreciate is that the stress parents feel and exhibit around their child's eczema can actually worsen the eczema. We will explore the connection between stress and eczema in the next chapter.

Chapter Takeaways

- The high-calorie, low-micronutrient Western diet has led to a malnourishment epidemic—an obese population lacking essential vitamins and minerals.
- There are likely dozens of vitamin and mineral deficiencies that will ultimately be found to play a role in eczema, but I have found three to be the most common: vitamin D, zinc, and omega-3.
- If possible, obtain micronutrients from fresh fruits and vegetables, whole foods, organic meats, and wild-caught fish. However, if supplementation is necessary, be sure to use a reliable, third-party-tested supplement manufacturer.

For discounts on high quality supplements in my online store, scan the QR code below.

10

Don't Stress Out

Stress is probably the single most underappreciated cause of eczema. Increasingly, studies are showing the relationship between stress in individuals or families and its unfavorable health effects.[116] In 1998, a severe cold snap hit the Canadian provinces of Quebec and Ontario. A succession of ice storms caused power outages to nearly 600,000 people during some of the coldest weeks of the year. The power was out for many weeks. Hundreds of thousands of families were temporarily displaced to emergency shelters.

This unfortunate situation gave scientists an interesting research opportunity.[117] Given the sheer number of people affected, a large number of women happened to be pregnant at the time. This allowed scientists to compare these women to women living in the same area who conceived and carried children without a stressful evacuation.

A number of studies were born out of this unique situation. One of the key elements observed in babies who were carried

---

[116] https://www.ncbi.nlm.nih.gov/pmc/articles/PMC5137920/

[117] https://www.mcgill.ca/projetverglas/icestorm

during this time was a change in their DNA. The stress of the ice storm on their mothers actually changed the babies' genetics. Many of these changes were a result of the inflammation that accompanies maternal stress.

> **The stress of the ice storm on their mothers actually changed the babies' genetics.**

As the children grew, it was noted they were at increased risk for a number of diseases, particularly inflammatory diseases such as asthma and eczema, as well as cognitive and learning deficiencies. The long-term effects on children induced by these stressful events during pregnancy has been called prenatal maternal stress (PNMS) syndrome. It appears that stress begins to play a role in eczema development from the moment of conception.

Stress in Parents

I have seen so many expecting mamas in my clinic who are stressed out of their minds and worrying about every aspect of their pregnancy—childbirth, body image, work, social media, finances, and a host of other things. The problem is that our brains don't differentiate between a saber-toothed tiger that wants to eat us for lunch and an overdue work project. Both things trigger an area of our brain, the hypothalamus, which stimulates the production of cortisol, also known as the stress hormone.

Cortisol gets us ready for fight or flight, shifting resources away from non-vital functions to urgently needed actions for survival. Things like higher heart rate, breathing capacity, muscle energy, and vision are prioritized over food digestion and the immune system. There's not much use in fighting a virus or bacteria that may take weeks to kill us when a violent death is staring us in the face. This chronic dysregulation of the immune system, modulated by cortisol, puts us at risk for eczema in several ways.

Cortisol is an immune system regulator. Excess cortisol causes an imbalance in the body's immune responses. As a result, it sends out molecules that promote inflammation. Our bodies then ramp up production of immunoglobulin E (IgE) antibodies and cause allergic reactions.

The body also experiences various other physiological changes that affect the skin. For example, the production of histamine-carrying mast cells increases. (We discuss the role of histamines in eczema in Chapter 8.) Stress also causes our blood vessels to dilate, which leads to a further release of histamine. Additionally, sensory nerves release molecules that can disrupt the normal functions of the outermost layer of the skin (aka, the skin barrier). These and other responses work in concert during stressful events and drive eczema symptoms.

In pregnancy, cortisol easily crosses the placenta, bombarding the fetus with stress hormones and preparing the baby for attack. Unfortunately, persistent exposure to high levels of cortisol alters the baby's immune system.

So, what if the pregnancy and delivery are all rainbows and unicorns but the maternal stress begins after birth? Unfortunately, the same thing occurs.

Studies have found that when parents are significantly stressed during their child's first few years of life, some of the children's genes involved in insulin production and in brain development are affected even years later, in adolescence.[118, 119] The

[118] https://developingchild.harvard.edu/wp-content/uploads/2005/05/Stress_Disrupts_Architecture_Developing_Brain-1.pdf

[119] https://www.ncbi.nlm.nih.gov/pmc/articles/PMC3202072/

changes in the brain caused by stress are not only hormonal—they can also be genetic, or epigenetic, which is the study of how genes can be turned on or off by certain environmental cues, stress being one of them (see Chapter 3).

Stress Begets Stress

Not only does parental stress contribute to the development of childhood eczema, but it also increases the risk of lifelong stress in the child. The genes in question are altered through a process called methylation. In a famous study, McGill University researcher Michael Meaney found that rats that spent significant amounts of time grooming and licking their pups had pups that were much calmer and more exploratory than their counterparts who got little to no grooming. This was accompanied by changes in their DNA. Interestingly, when the neglected pups were placed with foster mothers that groomed and licked them, their DNA transformed to look like that of the well-cared-for animals.[120]

In the rat world, grooming and licking is the hallmark of a low stress environment. Humans don't groom and lick their children to lower stress (at least not the licking!), but parents definitely set the stress level of the home. Our children's brains (and DNA) actually change as a response to their stressed-out parents. These brains then produce stressed-out kids who go on to perpetuate the cycle with their own children.

Another persuasive argument for the subtly harmful effect of parental stress on kids is what's called *heart-brain synchronization*. An electromagnetic field (EMF) is created by the heart as it beats. (This is what we measure when we perform an EKG on someone having a heart problem.) The interesting thing is

---

[120] https://pubmed.ncbi.nlm.nih.gov/16262207/

that our brain's electromagnetic field changes as the heart's EMF varies. Even more astonishing, the brains of people we touch or are close to will also change based on variation in our heartbeats.

Studies have confirmed that when I am stressed, the brains of those around me will synchronize to my stress level.[121] Thus, our children are incredibly sensitive to changes in our general stress level, and this is even more pronounced in utero. When you add stress in a parent or child to the myriad other factors described in this book, you have created the perfect eczema storm.

But your child's skin isn't the only thing that will suffer under the weight of stress in the home.

Side Effects of Stress

Hopefully, I have convinced you that we are largely responsible for instigating the stress response in our children. Worse still is that ongoing stress in a child can cause or exacerbate a number of issues, including:

- Skin and hair problems (such as acne, psoriasis, and eczema) and permanent hair loss
- Mental health problems, such as depression, anxiety, and personality disorders
- Cardiovascular disease, including heart disease, high blood pressure, abnormal heart rhythms, heart attacks, and stroke
- Obesity and other eating disorders
- Menstrual problems and fertility issues
- Sexual dysfunction, such as impotence and premature ejaculation in men, and loss of sexual desire in both men and women

---

[121] https://www.nature.com/articles/s41593-017-0044-6

- Gastrointestinal problems, such as gastroesophageal reflux disease (GERD), gastritis, ulcerative colitis, and IBS

Our culture is so inundated with stress, many of us don't even realize it has become our new baseline. Ask yourself these questions:

- Do I take sleep medications?
- Do I take anxiety medications?
- Am I snappy?
- Am I on edge?
- Do I blow up easily?
- Do I need a drink in the early evening to deal with life?
- Do I have a drink in the evenings so the kids are less annoying, or to calm myself?
- Do I have a need to constantly move and be productive?
- Do I eat a spectacular diet but still feel fluffy around the middle?

If you answered yes to two or more of these questions, you are likely experiencing increased stress. Let's work on getting that stress under control.

Cut Down Screen Time to Reduce Stress

So, what is the antidote to all this stress? Let's start with the low-hanging fruit—our phones. American adults spend an average of ten and a half hours on screens per day. Three and a half hours of that is on our mobile devices,[122] which give off elec-

[122] https://www.nielsen.com/us/en/insights/report/2016/the-total-audience-report-q1-2016/

tromagnetic radiation that activates your brain—*even when the phone is not in use!*

> *Devices give off electromagnetic radiation that activates your brain—even when the phone is not in use!*

Harvard University researchers placed participants in a brain scanner along with cell phones that were either switched off or on, but not functioning.[123] Participants did not know if the phones were off or on, as they were silenced. When the phones were switched on, the participants showed increased glucose (sugar) uptake in the brain. Thus, our phones are occupying our brains even when we are not actively using them! And to make matters worse, our phones are now attached to our wrist (hello, Apple Watch).

The most obvious take-home point for me from this study is that we must get phones out of the bedroom. First of all, if the phone is on the nightstand, we are more likely to use it at night, increasing our exposure to blue light and negatively impacting our sleep (another cause of stress). Secondly, even if we are not using them, the phones are still activating our brains. Take note: airplane mode is NOT good enough because Bluetooth and Wi-Fi still signal the brain. If it can't be out of the room, it should be powered off completely.

Next, notifications on your phone should be turned off. Each time we get a notification, it takes us approximately 23 minutes to return to the task at hand.[124] This is particularly true for social

---

[123] https://jamanetwork.com/journals/jama/fullarticle/645813

[124] https://www.ics.uci.edu/~gmark/chi08-mark.pdf

media notifications, as these often take us down the rabbit hole of an Instagram feeding frenzy (my personal weakness).

News apps can be even worse. Many of us are now attached to our phones, so we can get the latest and greatest news of doom and gloom about pandemics, wars, and the economy. This kind of news has upped the ante on stress. The old journalism adage "If it bleeds, it leads" is pure poison for our stressed-out brains.

Last, the best way to reduce the stress related to your child's eczema is to join my online community and program. Having experts lead the way, helping you with the dos and don'ts of gut healing, food replacements, and supplement dosing, will reduce your cortisol levels and the hours you spend on Google. Anxiety and stress play such a huge role in eczema that we have entire modules dedicated to this, and mental health is addressed on every live call.

The Busyness Badge

I used to wear my busyness as a badge of honor. When asked, "How are you doing?" by a friend, I responded proudly, "Been really busy." In fact, I don't think I've ever heard a mom respond, "You know, I'm so stressed and exhausted that I just sat on the couch all day and watched Netflix."

A friend of mine has three children who are all severely overscheduled. Recently, she was complaining that she couldn't figure out a way to fit piano practice between her son's football and soccer practices. One of her solutions was to feed the other kids dinner in the car while driving between practices to "free up some time." I told her she was nuts and that the rational thing to do would be to drop a few activities—but as I thought about it, I realized that this was me for many years. I sacrificed homemade meals and fed my kids fast food chicken nuggets—or worse—in the car to free up some time.

We think we are creating well-rounded kids with all these activities, but we are really molding stressed-out children who will end up resenting us for forcing them to participate in every sport, dance, instrument, club, or committee under the sun. And you now know that those stressed-out kids grow up to be stressed adults and perpetuate the cycle.

While I am at it, we mothers need to get better at outsourcing. Kids should be doing dishes and other chores, even if they do a crappy job—get over it! (I mean this in the nicest way possible.) Hire nieces/nephews and neighborhood kids to help out with babysitting, homework, grocery shopping, and so forth. There is no medal of honor awarded to the busiest mom of the year. Remember, it was the rats that took their time grooming and licking their pups that fared best, not the ones that had each pup in five types of gymnastics.

Try to master the art of single-tasking. Studies have shown that multitasking is actually a pipe dream; the human brain functions poorly while performing multiple tasks.[125] So, put your phone away while playing with your child, turn off your electronic device when your spouse or child walks into the room after work or school, help with homework after you've cooked dinner rather than during meal prep, eat dinner seated as a family, and watch your children thrive.

Social media can be particularly stress-inducing for our adolescent children. Any embarrassing social miscue that was once seen only by a few is now potentially seen by thousands—with catastrophic reputation and self-worth implications. Limiting time on social media, particularly before bed, can help. Start by

---

[125] https://academic.oup.com/hcr/article-abstract/42/4/599/4064731?redirectedFrom=fulltext

talking to your teens about the unrealistic standards on social media and educating them that self-worth is not derived from "likes" online but from real relationships. Last, be the role model for your child on social media.

Remember the Canadian women we discussed at the beginning of the chapter who were caught in the terrible ice storm in 1998? What I didn't tell you is that researchers are still studying their kids and finding more problems as they get older. In contrast to those women who had no control over a freak weather phenomenon, we have control over many of the stresses in our lives.

Could you and your child be at risk from the toxic effects of stress? If yes, you are not a bad parent, and you are not doomed. You are like the rest of us, trying to do the best you can. But maybe the best thing you can do is simply say "No." Your child's skin will thank you.

This topic is so important, I address it every week on our live calls during our Eczema Transformation group visit. The parents have seen huge benefits in their families' lives and their children's skin—just by implementing one simple mindset change at a time.

In addition to the stress our brains encounter while dealing with eczema and busy lives, our skin is feeling the pressure too. In the next chapter, we will look at some of the unique stresses skin must undergo when dealing with eczema.

Chapter Takeaways

- Chronic stress increases our levels of circulating cortisol, a stress hormone that disrupts the normal function of our immune system and places us at risk of autoimmune disease.

- The effects of stress begin in the womb and continue through childhood, causing changes in our DNA and resulting in increased incidences of eczema and other disorders.
- Start stress reduction with less exposure to screens (mobile phones), and by optimizing sleep and reducing scheduled activities.

To work with our mindset coaches on stress, go to our book resources page by scanning the QR code below.

11

Getting Under Your Skin

Medicine can be terribly humbling at times, particularly when treating children's eczema. But my most humbling patient experiences have taught me the most about managing this frustrating disease.

I want to tell you Tyler's story, as it provides a wonderful picture of how both the skin and gut play a role in eczema.

Tyler first came to see me as a gangly 8-year-old who had suffered from eczema for years. Her parents, Mark and Stacy, had tried all the traditional treatments, including topical creams and steroids, eliminating dairy, antihistamines, oral steroids, and more.

I was confident Tyler still had a sick gut, so my first order of business was to heal it. After about four months of dietary changes, lifestyle adjustments, stress management, and a supplement and probiotic regimen to resolve her deficiencies, she still had red, inflamed patches of itchy skin and showed minimal improvement. Many of her eczema lesions had become intermittently infected, with pus on top of the redness.

Mark and Stacy were highly concerned over the infected lesions and couldn't understand why our management hadn't seemed to help. Stacy brought Tyler to the office one day to show me the infected areas. "It just keeps getting worse and worse," Stacy exclaimed. Tyler just sat there quietly, trying not to scratch her elbows. As I examined her arms, I saw that she had large red areas of weeping eczema with pus and drainage from multiple areas. It looked horrible.

Have you ever been in a situation where you did everything "by the book" but still were not getting the result you wanted? Did you double down on what you were already doing to see if trying harder would work? I clearly needed to try something different with Tyler, but I wasn't sure in which direction I should head.

New Directions

As I pondered Tyler's weeping skin, it reminded me of some high school football players I had seen who had developed antibiotic-resistant staph infections in the locker room. Tyler had never been in sports, nor had she been exposed to known MRSA infections at school. I began to research skin infections in eczema, and it opened my eyes to a whole new aspect of the disease: the skin microbiome.

Our skin is the largest organ in our body. If you count all the dips, holes, and crevices for hair follicles and sweat glands, it actually has a surface area of more than 25 square meters (roughly the floor space of a two-car garage). That entire surface is covered in bacteria, viruses, fungi, and mites—YIKES.

The skin provides a vital physical barrier, protecting our bodies from assault by foreign organisms or toxic substances. But it is also an interface for our immune system to interact with bacteria that provide important functions—just like in our guts. For example, many of these bacteria interact with our white blood cells, teaching them which bacteria to tolerate and which to attack.

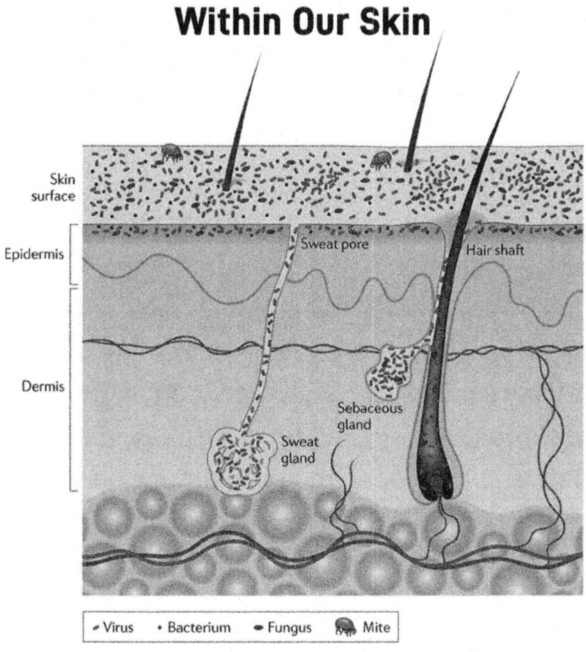

Figure 11.1

While we are in the womb, our skin is sterile; it becomes colonized by microorganisms only as we pass through the birth canal. This is another reason vaginal birth is so important; not only is our gut microbiome established in the vaginal canal, but our skin microbiome is too. The skin microbiome develops over the first year of life but is constantly changing, based on what's happening in our body, on our skin, and in our environment. Skin cells are replenished every 14 days in a baby and every 28 days in an adult. So microorganisms and our skin are engaged in a constant tango of acceptance or denial, based on the microorganism in question.

The organisms on our skin are also very picky about where they choose to call home. The living environment in our armpits is very different than on our knees (just smell any teenage boy).

Specific bacteria capitalize on these differences. Little holes and folds in our skin (called *invaginations* and *appendages*)—including sweat glands (*eccrine* and *apocrine*), sebaceous glands, and hair follicles—are associated with their own unique microorganisms as well.

The characteristic smell of sweat is created when apocrine sweat glands, located in the armpits and groin, interact with bacteria in those areas. The resulting waste products have a sulfur-like odor. Similar types of bacterial/skin interactions continuously occur all over our bodies in an attempt to maintain a steady state. Just like in our guts, some of the biggest balancing acts are between beneficial and problematic bacteria.

Staph Meeting

You have probably heard of a staph infection. More than 45 species of *staphylococcus* have been discovered, with more likely to come. Two specific *staphylococcus* species wage continuous war on our skin for control of the territory: *Staphylococcus aureus* (*S. aureus*) and *Staphylococcus epidermidis* (*S. epidermidis*).

S. epidermidis is a typically "friendly" bacteria on our skin that helps train our white blood cells. Cells in our skin (called keratinocytes) continuously sample the local bacteria to determine whether they are dangerous. If they are deemed harmful, the skin cells initiate an inflammatory response and produce proteins that can kill the bacteria.

Our skin is amazingly good at figuring out which bacteria to keep and which to attack. Although we don't completely understand why, evidence exists that *S. epidermidis* is a major player in helping the skin perform the evaluation process.[126] *S. epidermidis* not only directly blocks the growth of *S. aureus* and other dangerous species, but it also aids the proteins our skin cells make to kill the bad staph. Last, *S. epidermidis* can help calm down our skin's immune response when it becomes too active.

S. aureus plays the villain in this battle and clearly has a role in eczema lesions. More than 90 percent of eczema patients are colonized with *S. aureus* on both affected and non-affected skin, compared with less than 5 percent of healthy individuals. Additionally, eczema patients have lower levels of bacteria-fighting proteins produced by their skin cells, and *S. aureus* takes advantage of the situation.

Another problem with *S. aureus* is that it secretes an enzyme to break down ceramide. Ceramides are lipids (a type of fat molecule) that are found naturally in our skin (Figure 11.2). They're the body's built-in moisturizer. They make up the majority of the stratum corneum—the top layer of skin—and are responsible for holding the cells together.

In addition to acting as the glue that keeps the skin barrier intact, ceramides are moisturizing agents that make skin feel soft. Of note, ceramides make up much of the white, cheese-like substance (vernix) found coating the skin of newborn infants. By breaking down ceramide, *S. aureus* can disrupt the protective skin barrier, allowing it to enter our body. The breakdown of ceramide also leads to loss of moisture and subsequent changes in pH. And, as it turns out, pH is pretty important to our skin.

---

[126] https://journals.plos.org/plospathogens/article?id=10.1371/journal.ppat.1009026

Ceramide and Our Skin

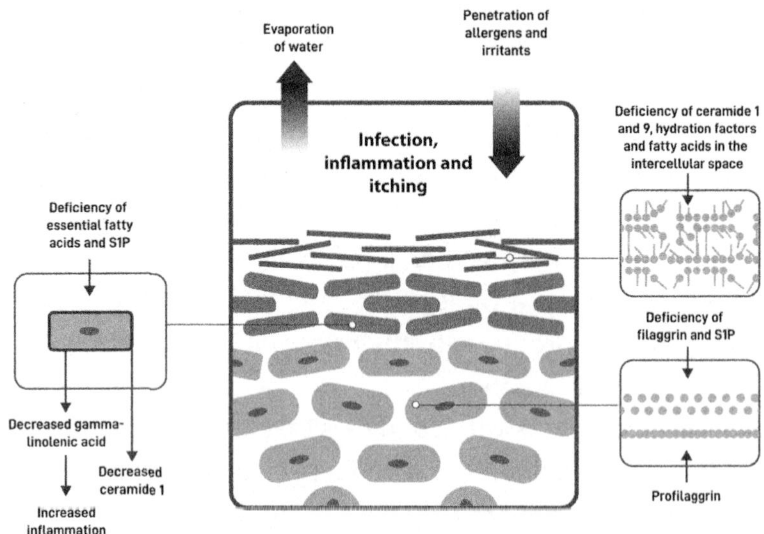

Figure 11.2

Don't Be Basic

Back to a little basic chemistry here: pH determines if something is more acidic (pH below 7) or basic (pH above 7). Water is neutral, with a pH of 7 (see Figure 11.3 for the pH of other common substances). Newborn skin begins with a neutral pH, and the transition to acidity begins in the first year of life. The greatest changes occur in the first two months. Of note, pH changes go from more acidic to more basic in the elderly, in part due to a ceramide deficiency that occurs with aging.

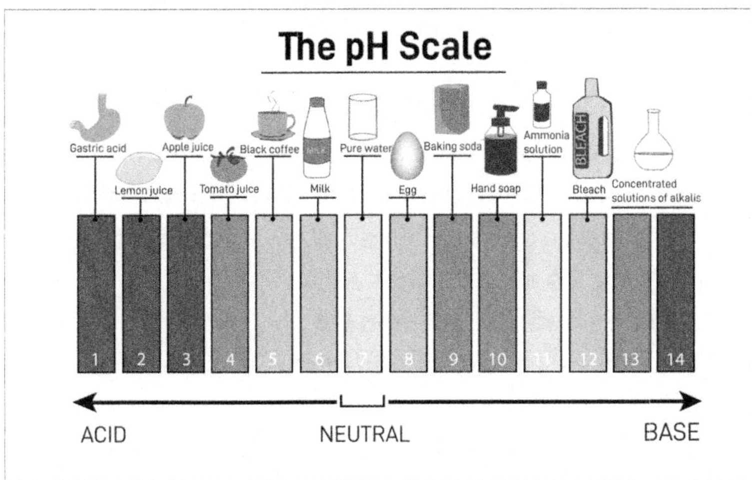

Figure 11.3

Although ceramide is important for maintaining acidic skin pH, its counterpart, filaggrin, is even more critical. You may remember filaggrin from the genetics section of Chapter 3, where I discussed a defect in the filaggrin gene that is known to increase the risk of eczema. In addition to providing strength to the skin barrier and holding in moisture, filaggrin induces the release of amino acids, which causes the skin to become more acidic. Guess who hates growing in an acidic environment? Yep, *S. aureus*. The skin's antimicrobial properties are optimal at acidic pH ranges, typically in the 4 to 5 range. This is one of our natural defense mechanisms, as many of the harmful bacteria on our skin can't tolerate a pH that low.

Many other factors can affect pH, though. Body site plays a role in skin pH, with infants experiencing higher levels on extensor surfaces and prominences, such as cheeks and buttocks. Children continue having a higher pH on surfaces such as inner elbows, wrists, ankles, and behind the knees. Later, in normal adult skin, the intertriginous zones (between fingers and toes) tend to have the highest pH.

> **Acidic pH is critical to the overall function of the skin.**

A lot of things can disrupt our skin's natural pH and break down the acid mantle. Factors such as what kind of products we put on our skin, the kinds of foods we eat, soaps and other topical products, sun and UV exposure, smoking, drinking, and many other things can disrupt the way the skin protects itself. Our diet, in particular, plays an important role in determining our internal pH and the pH levels of our skin. Acidic pH is critical to the overall function of the skin. *Staphylococcus* and other pathogenic bacteria love neutral pH and cannot work properly in an acidic environment.

Barrier Damage

I discussed the concept of the leaky gut and its relationship to eczema at length in Chapter 4. A leaky gut allows foreign materials to pass between intestinal cells and encounter the bloodstream. Our immune cells encounter these unwelcome invaders and mount a massive immune response.

To draw a comparison, the skin barrier in eczema also becomes leaky. Normally, skin cells and skin proteins, including ceramide and filaggrin, create a watertight barrier to carefully control what enters our bodies. Specialized white blood cells are able to reach through the tight barrier—without affecting their integrity—and "feel" the bacteria to determine if they are friend or foe. In eczema, these tight junctions are compromised, allowing bacteria to move deeper into our skin layers. The gaps also allow water to escape, further hampering the normal function of the skin.

A leaky skin barrier alone is not enough to cause eczema, but it is another factor to add to the inflammatory bucket. Even patients who are not able to maintain a normal barrier because of a severe genetic defect in filaggrin may never develop eczema if they have kept their immune systems in check. Other factors must contribute to the complex process.

We are just beginning to understand many of the complex interactions between microorganisms and our skin. It is clear that these interactions are altered in disease states. It also brings into question so many of the products we use in daily life. The antibacterial soaps, cleansing agents, and numerous chemicals we wield to "kill germs" have deleterious effects on our skin.

The antibacterial soaps, cleansing agents, and numerous chemicals we wield to "kill germs" have deleterious effects on our skin.

We have known for years that fastidiously clean households have a higher incidence of atopic diseases like allergic rhinitis, eczema, and asthma. This reinforces the adage that perhaps the best thing you can do for your kids is to let them play in the dirt or on the floor of the New York City subway, to build healthy skin biomes before eczema appears.

Decoding Topicals

In addition to the dozens of cleaners and other harmful agents our skin encounters each day, most families I have treated for eczema are applying numerous topical agents. The global skin-care market topped $145 billion in 2020, and those numbers are rising steadily.[127] You can bet that the big skin care product manufacturers are cashing in on ending the Eczema Epidemic, with promises of beautiful skin and eczema relief. Families attempting to decipher the topical eczema treatment puzzle are confused and stressed by the sheer number of products. The reality is that no one person's eczema etiology (set of causes) is the same. As a result, there is no one-size-fits-all topical eczema product.

To make things easier, I like to break down topical treatments into several broad categories, based on their primary function. However, there is often significant overlap between products, as some may moisturize *and* have anti-inflammatory properties. The lists below are not meant to be comprehensive; there are literally thousands of topical products marketed to the eczema community.

I favor natural products that don't have systemic effects. Additionally, the goal is not to crush our natural immune system but rather to relieve symptoms while we heal from the inside.

The list below has been compiled to inform you of what is out there, not necessarily what I recommend.

Anti-inflammatory topicals

- **Prescription Medications:** Topical steroids (hydrocortisone), phosphodiesterase 4 (PDE4) inhibitors (Eucrisa), topical calcineurin inhibitors (TCIs) (Tacrolimus), JAK inhibitors (Opzelura)

---

[127] https://www.researchandmarkets.com/reports/5141056/cosmetic-skin-care-global-market-trajectory-and?utm_source=GNOM&utm_medium=PressRelease&utm_code=xb4nlw&utm_campaign=1443716+-+Global+Cosmetic+Skin+Care+Industry+(2020+to+2027)+-+Market+Trajectory+%26+Analytics&utm_exec=jamu273prd

- **Natural Options:** Calendula, St. John's wort, zinc pastes, coconut oil, sunflower oil, colloidal oatmeal, primrose oil, blackseed oil

Antimicrobial topicals

- **Prescription Medications:** Topical antibiotics (Mupirocin, Neosporin)
- **Natural Options:** Manuka oil, coconut oil, baking soda, aloe vera, colloidal silver

Moisturizers

- **Ointments and Oils:** Highest oil content; includes petroleum jelly, mineral oils, emu oil, jojoba oil
- **Creams:** Less oil than ointment; many include ceramide skin barrier
- **Lotions:** Lowest oil content; often contain additional ingredients like alcohol, which may cause irritation

pH Balancers

- Alpha-hydroxy acids (citric acids, glycolic acids), hypochlorous acid (SkinSmart, Force of Nature), apple cider vinegar

Baths

- Colloidal oatmeal bath
- Bentonite clay
- Oil bath (coconut)
- Salt bath
- Apple cider vinegar bath
- Bleach bath

I want to emphasize, again, that topicals have value for short-term relief of symptoms and skin microbiome rebalancing.

However, I do *not* think topicals are the long-term solution to healing eczema. Any advertisements touting the miracle cure cream or ointment for eczema should be judged with skepticism. If families invested half the amount of money in whole foods and nontoxic products that they spend on topical agents, I would not need to write this book.

If families invested half the amount of money in whole foods and nontoxic products that they spend on topical agents, I would not need to write this book.

In my Eczema Transformation Program, I suggest topicals based on the current eczema symptom of the child. If dryness and itching are significantly impacting family life, I may use emu oil and zinc oxide as a skin barrier. (You can get my free guide to preferred holistic eczema creams by scanning the QR code at the end of the chapter.)

It's important to note that there is no cookbook solution to topicals, as some kids cannot tolerate certain agents. If weeping and pus are present, I may need to use a topical antibiotic to curb the infection and rebalance the skin microbiome. This was the case with Tyler, the young lady I introduced at the beginning of this chapter.

I believe Tyler had a major imbalance in her skin microbiome, so we began attempts to normalize the ratio of good to bad bacteria in her skin. First, we looked at any environmental agents at her home that would alter her skin pH: detergents, soap, toothpaste, countertop cleaners, sunscreen, bug spray, plug-in air fresheners, water, indoor air quality, and dust mites. I then needed to use an antimicrobial agent on her skin to reduce the amount of *S. aureus* and allow the good bacteria to repopulate.

There are several options to control a topical infection, and oral antibiotics are not needed in most cases. (If your child has a skin infection, please speak with your doctor about appropriate treatment.)

Since Tyler's infection was moderate to severe, I put her on a prescription topical antimicrobial protocol, while using a hypochlorous acid formulation to reduce the pH of the skin and further reduce bacterial counts. As her skin healed, I weaned her off the prescription medication, continued the hypochlorous acid, and added a skin rebalancing cream. In just over two months, her skin cleared up. This lovely young girl helped me dig deeper into other causes of eczema and develop more comprehensive protocols to address the skin microbiome. This case also reminded me of the premise of holistic care—treating the whole person, inside and out.

Chapter Takeaways

- The skin provides a vital physical barrier, protecting our bodies from assault by foreign organisms or toxic substances. But it is also an interface for our immune system to interact with bacteria that provide an important function (a microbiome, just like in our guts).
- Genetic defects in skin proteins, loss of ceramide, abnormal pH, and damage to the skin microbiome all contribute to skin barrier damage and the development of eczema.
- Natural topical treatments have value for short-term relief of symptoms and skin microbiome rebalancing, but I do not think topicals are the long-term solution to healing eczema.

A list of my current favorite topicals for eczema relief can be found at our book resources page by scanning the QR code below.

12

Putting It All Together

By now, many of you may have already embarked on your eczema healing journey. My hope is that you now understand that eczema is more than skin-deep. It represents a complex condition with a runaway immune system at its core. Our immune systems are waging a constant losing battle with the food industry, Big Pharma, environmental pollutants, stress and anxiety, and all the other inflammatory contributors we have discussed in this book.

We examined all the misconceptions circulating about eczema, including its origins, causes and triggers, treatments, and prognosis. The old adage "Kids will outgrow eczema" is a misnomer—more than 20 percent of kids will suffer eczema flares into adulthood.

We looked at the central role diet plays in the development of eczema. Food sensitivities tend to be the major culprit in eczema inflammation, rather than overt food allergies, which are often the focus of Western medicine. Food allergy and food sensitivity testing are different modalities examining two sides of the immune system: one related to life-threatening anaphylactic reactions and the other related to long-term immune tolerance.

However, elimination (replacement) diets remain the gold standard for determining food sensitivities. As food sensitivities activate inflammatory pathways of our immune system, many other factors are contributing to our inflammatory buckets.

Every person maintains a certain amount of inflammation that they can tolerate or hold—which I call their inflammatory bucket. As factors such as diet, medications, environmental toxins, genetics, and stress add to the inflammatory bucket, the bucket overflows. However, none of these factors on their own are enough to cause eczema. This is the entire premise behind autoimmune disorders, which have become rampant in industrialized nations. One of the major factors that many industrialized nations seem to share is the Western diet.

By understanding how our bodies evaluate and process the food we eat, we can better understand how our diets relate to autoimmune disease. Both maternal and children's diets are integral to shaping gut health, with poor dietary choices leading to a sick or "leaky" gut. The leaky gut begins the inflammatory cascade that manifests on our skin as eczema. It also disrupts the normal microbiome, which represents an important part of our immune system. Healing the gut is absolutely imperative to the long-term healing of eczema.

Healing the gut is absolutely imperative to the long-term healing of eczema.

Our bodies contain many more bacterial cells than human cells, and evolution has created a wonderful symbiosis between the two. Our microbiomes are not only integral to our immune systems but also affect our brain function, help digest our food, protect against other bacteria that cause disease, and produce numerous vitamins. The rampant over-prescribing of antibiotics in medicine and the overuse of antibiotics by the food industry are damaging our microbiomes. But there is also a much more insidious insult to our microbiomes: sugar.

We reviewed how skyrocketing sugar intake in the Western diet overwhelms our microbiome, while also causing an obesity epidemic, increasing diabetes, and worsening our skin, to name only a few effects. Combined with processed foods, sugar was likely the leading cause of eczema in my own family.

We then learned about two specific food groups that are known to contribute to eczema development: dairy and gluten. A significant portion of the world is intolerant to dairy products, and it is no surprise that dairy is a culprit in eczema development. The proteins contained in cow's milk incite an inflammatory response in many humans, leading to overflows of the inflammatory bucket. Thus, temporary dairy replacement is always one of the first steps in setting up an eczema treatment regimen as we begin gut healing.

Gluten sensitivities are becoming more recognized as a source of inflammation. You now understand that gluten sensitivity is a more subtle cousin to gluten intolerance, otherwise known as celiac disease. The sheer amount of gluten in our diets—from breads to soups and salad dressings—has likely played a role in the sensitivity increase. Additionally, changes in the way wheat is grown has played a factor, with the overuse of pesticides such as glyphosate (Roundup) adding to our inflammatory levels.

In Chapter 8, we discussed the role histamines play in eczema development. Histamines are highly inflammatory molecules contained within mast cells, which are like piñatas floating around in our bodies. When the mast cells burst open, a massive inflammatory reaction occurs that may wreak havoc on our immune system. Some people either have mast cells that are too sensitive and break open to friendly substances, or have too much circulating histamine because they are deficient in the enzyme that cleans up the excess. In my experience, histamine overload is *not* the primary problem in most cases.

In the chapters on micronutrients, we discussed the importance of what I refer to as "the big three" of eczema: vitamin D, zinc, and omega-3. A significant portion of the world is low or deficient in one or more of these micronutrients, each of which has been linked to developing eczema. Correcting these deficiencies is an imperative step in the eczema healing journey. Ideally, these should be replenished through a diet of whole foods; however, we also learned that farming soil may be deficient in nutrients, leading to foods that are low in nutrients. Additionally, we spend much more time indoors and are not able to harness sunlight for vitamin D. Often, supplementation is required in addition to dietary or behavioral change.

Although dietary change and correcting the gut-skin immune axis is key to eczema management, the most overlooked contributor to eczema is stress. Persistent stress has a clear physiological effect on our body and skin. More importantly, stress in the parents appears to be just as important as stress in the child for creating these negative physiological effects, such as excessive cortisol production. Excessive cortisol production wreaks havoc on our immune system over time, increasing inflammation and reactivity in our skin. A dedicated plan to implement stress reduction practices for both parent and child are crucial to the success of our eczema transformation.

Finally, we reviewed skin factors that predispose us to eczema. I purposely left skin until the end, as I want to change the mindset of eczema as only a skin problem. It is truly a systemic issue. We learned that the skin has its own microbiome, much like our gut, and disturbance of the microbiome balance can predispose us to eczema. Additionally, factors such as pH, skin moisture, and the presence of certain proteins can play a role in eczema flares. The use of topicals to battle these flares is widespread and doesn't address the root cause of eczema. Although topicals may play a role in managing acute symptoms, they are not the solution to eczema relief.

The long-term solution to eczema is making the dietary, behavioral, and environmental changes in our lives that will not only optimize our immune system for wonderful skin but will also help in many other areas. I have traveled many eczema journeys with my own children and the thousands of children and adults I have treated. With that knowledge, I have created a better way to heal eczema that avoids toxic medications, steroids, and ineffective topicals. I have now made the program available to anyone with internet access as a step-by-step guide to implement the ideas set forth in this book.

We have created a loving community of like-minded families whose mission is to heal eczema in a nontoxic way. You can find more information by scanning the QR code below. I firmly believe that if we institute the ideas and regimens I present in this book and in my online program, we can end the Eczema Epidemic. I wish each of you the best of luck on your eczema healing journey and I would be honored to accompany you along the way.

We would love feedback from our readers! Questions or comments may be submitted on our book resource page by scanning the QR code below.

Resources

About The Eczema Pantry and The Eczema Kitchen

My name is Lindsay Kingdon, and I created The Eczema Pantry and The Eczema Kitchen. I am a mom of three boys and a health coach for the Eczema Transformation Program with Dr. Temple. I have a bachelor's degree from UNC-Chapel Hill and a culinary degree from Johnson & Wales University, with a professional background in catering and events.

Despite my culinary credentials and professional catering background, the bulk of my cooking recently has been for my boys and husband! My family's food journey has been a rocky road at times, largely driven by health issues related to our food choices. After suffering from skin issues, infertility, a miscarriage, postpartum depression, and anxiety, I realized I had gluten sensitivity and that our family consumed too much sugar and processed food.

A few years later, my second son developed eczema, and we were forced to once again examine our food choices as part of Dr. Temple's Eczema Transformation Program. As I transitioned my family to replacement foods, I began recording recipes to help other families like mine. My son's eczema completely healed, and our household has truly seen the power of food! Today, I help families navigate food substitutions and teach them how to incorporate more "food from the earth" (plants and clean animal products) into their diets. Given that experience, Dr. Temple invited me to become an integral part of the eczema program. So yes, I am one of the many success stories of Dr Temple's eczema program!

The Eczema Pantry and The Eczema Kitchen were created to help families promote healing through the food they consume.

The Eczema Pantry is meant to be used as a shopping guide to help you switch out your pantry products for fewer processed foods with lower levels of pesticides and inflammatory chemicals. Remember, this transition takes time, and you may not be able to incorporate all these changes at once. It is best to think of this as "replacement" rather than "elimination."

The Eczema Kitchen includes some allergy-friendly recipes for breakfast, lunch, dinner, and some household basics. These have all been tested in my home kitchen on my 9-, 5-, and 1-year-old sons, and my husband. It is vital to have doable, family-friendly recipes to get your whole family on board during this process!

Each recipe has a note under the title that lists the allergens it is free of, such as "gluten-free."

The Eczema Pantry

Produce

Ideally, try to transition to foods that have not been affected by Roundup (glyphosate). That is the main pesticide sprayed on produce, and it is dangerous to ingest. This swap does not have to happen overnight, but it is a good goal to work toward.

The Dirty Dozen is a list published online by the Environmental Working Group (EWG).[128] It is updated annually to include fruits and vegetables that are the most heavily affected by pesticides and herbicides, as well as the produce that is safe to buy non-organic. The lists below are based on the Dirty Dozen.

Buy organic for these foods:

- Strawberries
- Spinach
- Kale, collards, mustard greens
- Nectarines
- Apples
- Grapes

[128] https://www.ewg.org/foodnews/dirty-dozen.php

- Cherries
- Peaches
- Pears
- Bell and hot peppers
- Celery
- Tomatoes

Updated Dirty Dozen 2022 according to the EWG[129]

The following are usually okay to buy non-organic:

- Avocado
- Sweet corn
- Pineapple
- Onions
- Papaya
- Green peas (frozen)
- Eggplant
- Asparagus
- Broccoli
- Cabbage
- Kiwifruit
- Cauliflower
- Mushrooms
- Honeydew melon
- Cantaloupe

Meat and fish

The following is a list of ideal meat and fish that are a vital source of nutrients:

- Organic pasture-raised chicken
- Grass-fed beef

---

129 https://www.ewg.org/foodnews/dirty-dozen.php

- Wild-caught (not farmed) salmon
- Pasture-raised pork
- Lamb, turkey, duck, bison
- Beef or chicken liver

Eggs

Eggs can be an excellent source of nutrition. Buying ones from a farm where the chickens are able to roam on grass is ideal. Look for "pasture-raised" on the label in the grocery store, or purchase from a local farmers market. Pastured eggs or locally farmed eggs are best.

Egg replacements

The following options can replace one large chicken egg in a baking recipe.

- Option 1: Use 1 Tbsp ground flaxseed OR 1 Tbsp ground chia seeds + 3 Tbsp water. Leave it on the counter for 3 min. It will thicken up and become gelatinous.
- Option 2: Use 3 Tbsp aquafaba, which is the liquid from a can of chickpeas, or garbanzo beans.
- Option 3: Use ¼ cup of mashed banana or ¼ cup of unsweetened applesauce.

Nuts and seeds

In some people, nuts can be inflammatory and should be removed during the process of healing eczema. However, many people are able to eat the seeds listed below. They are a great source of fiber, fat, nutrients, and some protein.

- Raw pumpkin seeds
- Raw sunflower seeds
- Unsweetened coconut flakes
- Chia seeds

- Hemp seeds
- Ground flaxseed
- Raw almonds
- Raw cashews

Freezer items

- Frozen organic berries
- Frozen mango or pineapple
- Bone broth
- Allergy-friendly pie crust
- Cassava or almond flour tortillas
- Organic frozen veggies
- Gluten-free pizza crust

Dairy

Many plant-based and dairy-free milk options are filled with gums and other additives. A few brands have mainly nuts and water as their ingredients. Seed milks are also an option. Look for milk that is unsweetened with minimal ingredients.

Milk:

- Nut milk that is mainly nuts and water
- Oat milk, gluten-free organic oats
- Hemp, pumpkin, or flaxseed milk
- Coconut milk

Yogurt:

- Coconut milk yogurt, unsweetened
- Almond milk or cashew yogurt, unsweetened

Cheese:

Dairy-free cheese should not be relied on as a source of vital nutrients, but it is nice to have on hand for sandwiches and homemade pizza. Dairy-free cheese is often made with either soy, nuts, or coconut and potato starch.

Deli meat

Limit deli meat and bacon to a couple of times per week, and be careful because some types and brands contain sodium nitrites/nitrates, celery powder, added sugar and caramel color. Not all deli meat is gluten- and dairy-free, but you can check the brand's website to see the exact ingredients.

Oils

Each of the following oils have their own health benefits. Using a variety of the three is ideal. For baking, avocado oil can replace canola or vegetable oil in a recipe. Coconut oil is often used in gluten-free and paleo-style baking. Extra virgin olive oil is excellent for dressings, and for adding a good, healthy fat to a dish. For roasting vegetables, my preference is avocado oil, but any of the following three will work:

- Extra virgin olive oil
- Avocado oil
- Coconut oil

Vinegar

If histamines are a concern, **raw apple cider vinegar** is your best bet. The apple cider vinegar with "The Mother" contains probiotics that are great for gut health. This can be used in baking, marinades, and salad dressings.

Stock and wine for cooking

Stock and wine are sometimes needed for a recipe. Chicken or beef stock or broth should be made with bones, vegetables, water, and possibly herbs and spices. The Eczema Kitchen also has a recipe for how to make your own bone broth. If using wine in a recipe, organic is best.

Baking ingredients

The following are common ingredients for baking gluten-free recipes:

- Cassava flour
- Tapioca flour
- Finely ground almond flour
- Gluten-free flour blend
- Ground flax meal
- Arrowroot flour
- Aluminum-free baking powder
- Coconut flour
- Psyllium husk powder

Beans, legumes, pastas, and grains

Making the switch to gluten-free grains surprisingly offers more options than one might assume. Certain grains and legumes are naturally gluten-free, and they are listed below. Oats are not always gluten-free, so be sure to purchase oats, oatmeal, or granola that is properly labeled. The Eczema Kitchen has a recipe for homemade granola.

- Gluten-free pasta made from lentils, chickpeas, or quinoa
- Dried lentils
- Dried or canned beans
- Quinoa
- Rice*

- Cornmeal
- Gluten-free organic oats

*Many types of rice contain dangerously high levels of arsenic. To be safe, look for white rice, sushi rice from the U.S., and basmati rice from California, India, Pakistan. Avoid brown rice, unless it's from California, India, or Pakistan. (If you use brown rice, do so in limited amounts.) Also, avoid rice from Arkansas, Texas, Louisiana, and Bangladesh.

Sauces and condiments

Carefully read each ingredient list for sauces and condiments. Chapter 5 lists other types of sugar, and Chapter 7 lists sources of gluten and wheat.

- Gluten-free organic soy sauce
- Coconut aminos
- Avocado oil-based salad dressings
- Ranch dressing listed in The Eczema Kitchen
- Sugar-free organic ketchup
- Salsa
- Taco seasoning or homemade version
- Avocado oil mayonnaise
- Vegan mayonnaise (if it uses a healthy oil, like avocado)
- Sugar-free BBQ sauce
- Whole-grain mustard
- Raw honey
- Real maple syrup
- Raw apple cider vinegar

Keep a variety of mustards (Dijon, yellow, whole grain) on hand to combine with raw honey and raw apple cider vinegar for great marinades and sauces.

Packaged snacks

Look for snacks with as few ingredients as possible, and with ones you can pronounce. Snacks should have quality oils, as we are trying to avoid vegetable, seed, and canola oil. Chips and crackers can be cooked in avocado, olive, or coconut oil. At the minimum, buy products with organic sunflower oil.

The following is a list of the types of snacks that fit these criteria, but please be sure to read individual labels. Eating clean snacks 100 percent of the time is not always feasible, so we encourage you to limit snacks that do not meet this list to only once or twice per week.

- Chips, crackers, pretzels, popcorn (these should be cooked in avocado, olive, or coconut oil)
- Cassava flour tortilla chips
- Seed-based gluten-free crackers
- Almond crackers
- Flax crackers
- Gluten-free or grain-free pretzels
- Plantain chips
- Potato chips
- Unsweetened coconut chips
- Dried veggie chips
- Kale chips
- Seaweed crisps

Nuts should be raw or cooked in a healthy oil, like the ones mentioned above. Extra flavoring can potentially include sugar, gluten, or dairy, so raw or simply roasted nuts are the best option.

- Unsalted raw mixed nuts
- Nut butter squeeze packs
- Organic unsweetened applesauce packs

- Individual guacamole packs
- Individual hummus packs
- Olive snack packs
- Pickle snack packs
- Freeze-dried strawberries

Cereal

Look for cereals that are quite plain, gluten-free or grain-free, and with very little added sugar. Organic cereal is best, because some grains made for cereals are heavily sprayed with pesticides and herbicides. There is a gluten-free, nut-free granola recipe in The Eczema Kitchen. Store-bought granola should be sweetened with a minimal amount of honey, coconut sugar, or maple syrup.

For more recipes, including histamine-free meals, check out our book resource page by scanning the QR code below.

The Eczema Kitchen Recipes

One truth I've learned over the years, as we in our household have changed the way we cook and eat, is that food can still taste good even if it is allergy-friendly! Adjustments have to be made but there are lots of options to eat well. These recipes are family-friendly and have all been tested in my home kitchen. I have included a note at the top of each recipe to indicate whether it is free from any of the following: gluten, dairy, eggs, nuts, and soy.

Contents

Turkey or Beef Meatballs
Dairy-Free Macaroni and Cheese

Dinner:

Cedar-Planked Maple-Mustard Salmon
Lemon-Thyme Roasted Chicken
Grilled Steak Tacos with Guacamole
Dairy-Free Leek and Potato Soup

Side Dishes:

Ginger Asparagus
Roasted Carrots with Herbs
Cauliflower Mash
Mini Wedge Salads

Basics:

Dairy-Free Ranch Dressing
Hemp Milk
Oat Milk
Bone Broth
Pumpkin Seed Butter

Breakfast

Nut-Free Granola

Gluten-free, dairy-free, egg-free, nut-free, soy-free; coconut is optional

3½ cups gluten-free organic oats
½ cup hemp seeds*
½ cup chia seeds
½ cup ground flax seeds
1 cup raw sunflower seeds
1 cup raw pumpkin seeds
1 cup unsweetened coconut flakes
½ tsp sea salt
½ tsp cinnamon
½ cup coconut oil**
½ cup honey
½ tsp vanilla

Preheat oven to 300°F. In a large rimmed pan or casserole dish, mix together all of the dry ingredients (oats through cinnamon).

In a small pot on the stove, heat the coconut oil, honey, and vanilla until the coconut oil is melted. Drizzle the oil mixture over the oat and seed mixture. Use a heatproof spatula and stir it all together really well. Make sure to scrape the bottom of the pan with the spatula so that it is evenly incorporated.

Cook for 14 minutes, then remove from the oven and stir well. Repeat three times, for a total of four 14-minute cooking sessions. Remove from the oven and allow to cool before eating. It will crisp up as it cools.

*You could use all three seeds—hemp, chia, and flax—or just use 1½ cups of one kind. This recipe is flexible!

**You can use avocado oil instead of coconut oil. If you do, you can skip the step where you melt the coconut oil. Simply mix the liquid ingredients together without heating.

Apple Oat Muffins

Gluten-free, dairy-free, egg-free, nut-free, soy-free; does contain coconut
Makes 24 mini muffins

2 Tbsp ground flaxseed or flaxseed meal
6 Tbsp water
2 cups GF organic oats
7 dates, pitted
½ cup coconut oil, plus more for the pan, softened
⅛ tsp salt
1½ tsp cinnamon
1 tsp vanilla
2 apples, peeled and grated
1 tsp baking soda
½ tsp baking powder

Preheat the oven to 350°F. Grease a mini cupcake tin with coconut oil. In a small saucepan, stir together the water and flax. Heat over low heat for just a minute or two. Remove from the heat and allow to cool. Peel and grate the apples.

In a food processor or blender, add all of the ingredients. Pulse some, then scrape down the sides. Blend until the oats and dates have broken down and everything is in small pieces. It should be sticky, but not liquid.

Spoon the batter into the muffin tin, then bake for 15–18 minutes. Allow to cool for a few minutes, then remove from the muffin tin.

Tropical Green Smoothie

Gluten-free, dairy-free, egg-free, nut-free, soy-free
Makes 3–4 servings

¾ cup ice
1½ cups frozen mango
1½ cups frozen pineapple
2 handfuls baby kale or ¾ cup frozen organic kale
½ cucumber, chopped
1 inch ginger, peeled
½ lemon, juiced
4 dates
4 Tbsp hemp seeds
2 cups water, or as needed

Blend all ingredients together in a high-powered blender. Increase the speed as you go, and add water as needed.

Nut-Free Cassava Waffles

Gluten-free, dairy-free, nut-free, soy-free; egg-free option
Makes 10 waffles

1½ cups cassava flour
1 Tbsp baking powder
¾ tsp salt
1½ cups hemp milk or oat milk (see recipes), or other dairy-free milk
2 eggs
1 Tbsp maple syrup (optional)
2 Tbsp avocado oil

Preheat the waffle maker.

Whisk together the dry ingredients. Mix the wet ingredients in a separate bowl. Add the wet to the dry and mix well. Try to avoid lumps. The cassava flour tends to stick to the side of the bowl. Pour ¼–⅓ cup of batter into each square of the waffle maker. Cook until golden brown.

Nut-Free Pumpkin Oat Waffles

Gluten-free, dairy-free, nut-free, soy-free
Makes 10 waffles

1⅔ cups gluten-free oat flour
½ cup arrowroot powder
1 tsp cinnamon
½ tsp nutmeg
½ cup pumpkin puree (unsweetened)
¾ cup dairy-free milk (use hemp or oats to keep it nut-free)
¼ cup maple syrup
2 eggs*
3 Tbsp avocado oil
1 tsp vanilla
avocado oil spray

Preheat the waffle maker and spray it with the avocado oil spray.

Whisk together the dry ingredients. Mix the wet ingredients in a separate bowl. Add the wet to the dry and mix well. Try to avoid lumps.

Pour ⅓ cup of the batter into each square of the waffle maker. Cook until golden brown.

*See the egg substitution chart for alternatives. This recipe also works with flax "eggs."

Lunch

Chicken Nuggets

Gluten-free, dairy-free, egg-free, nut-free, soy-free; does contain coconut

1½ to 2 pounds chicken breasts, cut into 1½-inch pieces
1 cup cassava flour
⅓ cup coconut flour
2 tsp sea salt
⅛ tsp onion powder
½ tsp garlic powder
1 tsp paprika
¼ tsp black pepper
1 cup lite coconut milk
4 Tbsp avocado oil

Preheat oven to 400˚F. Line a baking sheet with parchment paper.

Pat the chicken pieces dry with paper towel. Pour the coconut milk into one shallow bowl. In another shallow bowl, mix the cassava flour, coconut flour, sea salt, onion powder, garlic powder, paprika, and black pepper.

Piece by piece, dip the chicken in the coconut milk, then dredge them in the flour mixture, then the coconut milk again, and the flour mixture again. Make sure to use lite coconut milk.

Lay the chicken pieces on the parchment paper-lined pan. Brush them carefully with avocado oil. Bake for 6 minutes, then flip over, and bake for another 6 minutes, or until the internal temperature of the chicken is at least 165˚F.

Allow to cool before refrigerating. These will be good for lunches for a few days. If they need to be crisped before adding them to a lunch box, use a toaster oven, or place in an oven preheated to 375°F for a couple of minutes. These can also be reheated in a sauté pan.

Turkey or Beef Meatballs

Gluten-free, dairy-free, egg-free, nut-free, soy-free

¼ cup grated onion
¼ cup grated carrot
½ tsp dried parsley
½ tsp dried oregano
½ tsp dried basil
2 Tbsp nutritional yeast
1¼ tsp kosher salt
1 tsp garlic powder
⅓ cup gluten-free oat flour
2 lb meat: grass-fed ground beef or organic ground turkey
1 Tbsp avocado oil if using turkey; no oil needed for beef
marinara, optional

Preheat the oven to 400°F. Line a rimmed baking sheet with parchment paper.

If using whole oats to make oat flour, pulse the oats in a food processor until ground. Wipe clean and then use the food processor to finely chop the onion and carrot.

Mix all the seasonings, vegetables, and flour. Then add the meat and gently mix in well. Form into small to medium meatballs and lay out evenly on the baking sheet. If using turkey, drizzle the meatballs with the avocado oil.

Bake for 20–25 minutes, rotating the pan halfway through. You can turn the meatballs halfway through if you prefer. These can be served with marinara sauce and pasta, or plain in a thermos for lunch.

Dairy-Free Macaroni and Cheese

Gluten-free, dairy-free, egg-free, soy-free, can be made nut-free

1 package GF chickpea or lentil pasta
2 Tbsp DF butter
2 Tbsp GF all-purpose flour
1½ cups DF milk, warmed
salt and pepper
⅛ tsp nutmeg
dash cayenne, optional
1 cup DF shredded cheese

Cook the pasta according to package directions, then drain.

Warm the dairy-free milk in a glass measuring cup in the microwave, or in a small saucepan on the stove. It just needs to be warm; do not bring to a boil.

In another pot, make the cheese sauce. Melt the dairy-free butter over low-medium heat. Whisk in the gluten-free flour and whisk constantly until blended well. After a minute, slowly add the milk that has been warmed, whisking constantly. The texture should be creamy, but not so thick that it is hard to stir, because it will continue to thicken. Season the sauce with salt, pepper, the nutmeg, and a dash of cayenne if you want a bit of spice. Stir well. Once it tastes right, stir in the shredded cheese. Make sure the heat is on low and stir with a heatproof spatula until the cheese is almost completely melted.

Stir in the cooked and drained noodles. To serve in a lunch box, make the macaroni and cheese ahead of time. Reheat the morning of and add to a thermos. This is great to serve with cooked chicken sausage and steamed broccoli.

Cedar-Planked Maple-Mustard Salmon

Gluten-free, dairy-free, egg-free, nut-free, soy-free

3 Tbsp whole-grain mustard
3 Tbsp maple syrup
2 Tbsp coconut aminos
2 Tbsp white wine vinegar
1 Tbsp chopped fresh rosemary
salt and pepper
1 to 1½ pounds wild caught Alaskan salmon
cedar plank (usually found near the fish counter at the grocery store)

Prep the salmon by checking for bones. Remove any pin bones that you find. Pat the salmon dry with paper towel. Soak the cedar plank in water for 30 minutes.

Mix the mustard, syrup, coconut aminos, vinegar, rosemary, salt, and pepper to taste. Pour ¾ of it over the salmon and allow the salmon to marinate for around 30 minutes.

Preheat the grill to medium heat, around 400°F.

Dry the cedar plank and place the salmon on it, skin side down. Carefully place the planks on the grill and cook for 7 minutes. Check the internal temperature of the salmon using a digital meat thermometer. Remove from the grill when the salmon is around 125–135°F.

Use the remaining marinade as a sauce and brush on the fish.

Dinner

Lemon-Thyme Roasted Chicken

Gluten-free, dairy-free, egg-free, nut-free, soy-free

1 whole organic (or local, pasture-raised) chicken
1 lemon, quartered
½ onion, chopped into 4 chunks
3 Tbsp olive oil
1½ Tbsp kosher salt
¾ tsp freshly ground pepper
8 fresh thyme sprigs

Remove the chicken from the plastic, take out any bags and so on from inside the chicken, and make sure to drain well. Place on an oven-safe roasting or cooling rack on top of a rimmed baking pan. Make sure the chicken is breast-side up. In a small dish, mix the salt and pepper. Preheat the oven to 400°F.

This may sound odd, but to achieve extra crispy skin, you can use your hairdryer to blow-dry the chicken; on the medium-heat setting, blow-dry the chicken for about three minutes.

Place the cut lemon and onion, along with half of the thyme, inside the cavity of the chicken. Drizzle the olive oil all over the chicken, and gently pull up the skin in some places to put the oil and seasonings there as well—under the skin, directly onto the meat. Next, sprinkle the salt and pepper on the outside, under the skin, and in the cavity. If it feels like too much salt and pepper, you do not have to use it all.

Optional: use kitchen twine to truss the chicken. The wing tips should be tucked underneath the legs, and the legs should be tied together. This step is not necessary, but it can help the chicken cook more evenly. For images, look for videos on YouTube.

Cook on the middle rack at 400˚F for 25 minutes. Then lower the temperature to 350˚F and cook for 25–30 minutes, or until each part of the chicken has an internal temperature of 165˚F. Use a digital meat thermometer, and make sure to check places other than just the breasts. Allow it to rest for 15 minutes before slicing.

Grilled Steak Tacos with Guacamole

Gluten-free, dairy-free, egg-free, nut-free, soy-free

grass-fed ribeye (2 steaks, or enough for 4 people)
2 bell peppers
1 sweet yellow onion
avocado oil
2–3 Tbsp taco seasoning
gluten-free corn tortillas
cilantro
dairy-free sour cream
guacamole (recipe below) or sliced avocado

Pat the steaks dry with paper towel. Cut the bell peppers and onion into wide slices. Rub a little avocado oil onto the steaks, and toss the peppers and onion slices in some avocado oil as well. Season the steak, peppers, and onion with the taco seasoning. Preheat the grill. Grill until the peppers and onion are lightly charred. Cook the steak to medium-medium rare. A digital meat thermometer should show an internal temperature of 135–145°F. Lightly grill some corn tortillas.

Allow the steak to rest for a few minutes after removing from the grill, then slice it thinly. To assemble the tacos, place a few pieces of pepper, onion, and steak onto each grilled tortilla. Garnish with dairy-free sour cream, cilantro leaves, and guacamole or avocado.

Guacamole

Gluten-free, dairy-free, egg-free, nut-free, soy-free

¼ cup yellow or sweet onion, diced small
1 small garlic clove, minced
1 tomato or 2 Roma tomatoes, seeds removed, diced small
½ jalapeño pepper, seeds removed, chopped small
handful cilantro, chopped
juice of ½ lime
¾ tsp sea salt
small pinch sugar
2–3 ripe avocados

Mix the first eight ingredients in a medium-sized bowl to make a pico de gallo. Taste and adjust accordingly. Add salt if needed. Add salt if needed. Then add the diced avocado and gently stir/mash with the back of a fork. If you prefer it to be mostly avocado, set aside some of the pico de gallo before adding the avocado.

Dairy-Free Leek and Potato Soup

Gluten-free, dairy-free, egg-free, nut-free, soy-free, contains coconut

3 Tbsp olive oil or dairy-free butter
2 whole carrots, diced small
2 stalks celery, diced small
1 larger leek, cleaned well, sliced in half, then chopped
3 lb red potatoes, peeled then chopped
4 cups bone broth, approximately
2–3 sprigs fresh thyme
1 bay leaf
salt and pepper
1½ cups coconut milk (canned)
bacon for garnish, optional

Heat the butter or olive oil in a large pot. Add the carrot, celery, and leeks, and sauté 5–8 minutes or until softened. Add the potatoes and sauté for a couple of minutes. Add the bone broth, thyme, and the bay leaf.

Stir, then bring to a boil and reduce to a simmer. Cook over low heat until the potatoes are soft. Add the milk. Season as needed with salt and pepper.

Purée the soup in a blender. Serve with crumbled bacon as a garnish.

Side Dishes

Ginger Asparagus

Gluten-free, dairy-free, egg-free, nut-free, soy-free

1 lb asparagus, ends trimmed
2 Tbsp olive oil or avocado oil
salt and pepper
½ tsp honey
½ inch fresh ginger, grated or minced

Heat a nonstick skillet over medium heat. Add the oil, then add the asparagus. Cook, stirring, for 7 minutes or until the asparagus are bright green. Add the ginger and cook for another minute. Season with salt and pepper and honey and cook for another minute, or until browned to your preference.

This is great to serve with the Cedar-Planked Maple-Mustard Salmon.

Roasted Carrots with Herbs

Gluten-free, dairy-free, egg-free, nut-free, soy-free

6 whole carrots, peeled
avocado oil
fresh chopped sage or thyme, or both
salt and pepper

Line a rimmed baking sheet with parchment paper. Chop the carrots in half, then into even (as best as you can) slices. If you have a wide section, cut it in half lengthwise, then in half again, to give you slightly thick spears.

Lay the carrots out evenly on the parchment-lined baking tray. Drizzle on some avocado oil, about 1 Tbsp, and gently toss the carrots in the oil. Sprinkle on the chopped herbs and salt and pepper. Roast at 375°F for 40 minutes.

Cauliflower Mash

Gluten-free, dairy-free, egg-free; can be nut-free depending on the milk used, and use olive oil instead of dairy-free butter

1 head cauliflower, cut into pieces, not too big
5 cups chicken stock*
2 garlic cloves, peeled
2 Tbsp dairy-free butter or extra virgin olive oil
½ cup unsweetened dairy-free milk, warmed
salt and pepper to taste

Place the cauliflower, garlic, and stock in a pot. *Use enough stock to just cover the cauliflower in a pot. Cover the pot and bring to a boil. Turn the heat down and boil lightly for 12 minutes, or until the cauliflower can be easily pierced with a fork.

Drain the liquid from the pot completely. Make sure all the liquid is out of the pot. Place the cooked cauliflower in a blender or food processor. Blend until puréed.

Add the olive oil or dairy-free butter and milk. Blend again until smooth. Season with salt and pepper as needed and blend again.

Mini Wedge Salads

Gluten-free, dairy-free

1 head iceberg lettuce
3 Roma tomatoes, diced small
6 slices of bacon, cooked and crumbled
3 green onions, chopped
¼ cup pecans, chopped and toasted
2 oz dairy-free feta
dairy-free ranch dressing (recipe below)
freshly cracked black pepper

Wash the iceberg lettuce and dry well. Chop the head of lettuce in half, then quarters, then into eighths, or even smaller into sixteenths. Lay them out into a casserole dish. Sprinkle each of the other ingredients evenly over the top of each wedge of lettuce. Then drizzle on the ranch dressing, and crack on some fresh black pepper.

Basics

Dairy-Free Ranch Dressing

Gluten-free, dairy-free

1 tsp dried parsley
½ tsp black pepper
1 tsp seasoning salt
½ tsp dried dill
½ tsp garlic powder
¼ tsp onion powder
⅛ tsp dried thyme
3 shakes cayenne powder (optional)
½ cup avocado oil mayonnaise
½ cup dairy-free sour cream
¼ cup dairy-free milk
¾ tsp apple cider vinegar

In a liquid measuring cup, mix the milk and vinegar and let sit for a few minutes. Mix the dry ingredients together in a bowl. Add the mayonnaise and the sour cream to the milk and whisk together. Then pour the spices into the liquid ingredients and whisk well. Allow to chill for an hour or so before serving. The flavor will develop.

Hemp Milk

Gluten-free, dairy-free, egg-free, nut-free, soy-free
Makes a little over 4 cups

½ cup shelled hemp hearts
2–3 pitted dates
a couple splashes of vanilla extract (optional)
4 cups filtered water

Blend all ingredients at medium speed, then turn the blender up to medium-high and blend until creamy. Strain through a nut milk bag or cheesecloth. Store in a glass jar and use within a week. Shake well before serving.

Oat Milk

Gluten-free, dairy-free, egg-free, nut-free, soy-free
Makes a little more than 3 cups

½ cup gluten-free organic oats
3 cups filtered water
pinch sea salt
2 dates (optional)
1 tsp maple syrup (optional)
½ tsp vanilla
(Sweeteners are optional.)

Blend all ingredients at medium speed. Then turn the blender up to medium-high and blend until creamy. Strain through a nut milk bag or cheesecloth. Make sure to twist the bag after the milk has strained most of the way through, to get all the creaminess. Store in a glass jar and use within a week. Shake well before serving.

Bone Broth

Gluten-free, dairy-free, egg-free, nut-free, soy-free

1 turkey or chicken carcass, or beef bones, most of the meat removed
(This can be bones that you've roasted and are left over, or bones you purchase from the butcher that have not been cooked. Please make sure the bones are from a good source, like grass-fed-beef bones)
12–14 cups filtered water, enough to cover the bones in the crock pot
2 Tbsp raw, unfiltered apple cider vinegar
3 stalks celery, large chop
2 large carrots, large chop
1 yellow (sweet) onion, large chop

Remove as much of the meat from the turkey or chicken carcass as possible. Place the carcass (bones) in a large crock pot. Add the celery, carrot, onion, and apple cider vinegar.

Carefully pour in the water. You need enough for the bones to be covered. Set the crock pot to low and cook for 18–24 hours.

Once the broth has cooked, you will need to strain it through a fine mesh strainer or sieve into a large glass (heatproof) bowl. Allow to cool, then store in mason jars in the refrigerator for up to a week. Broth can also be frozen in silicone soup cubes.

Pumpkin Seed Butter

Gluten-free, dairy-free, egg-free, nut-free, soy-free
Makes 1 to 1½ cups

2 cups sprouted or raw pumpkin seeds, unsalted
2 tsp avocado oil
½ tsp cinnamon
1½ tsp maple syrup
½ tsp vanilla extract
pinch salt

Preheat the oven to 350˚F. Spread the seeds out on a rimmed baking sheet and roast for 8 minutes. Allow the seeds to cool, then add them to a food processor. Blend the seeds for around 6–7 minutes, stopping every minute or minute and a half to scrape down the sides. The mixture will be crumbly, then a little sticky, then like a dough ball, and then it will become smooth and creamy. Add the flavorings and avocado oil and blend again for another 2–3 minutes. This can be stored at room temperature for a week, or in the refrigerator.

For more recipes including histamine-free meals, check out our book resource page by scanning the QR code below.

Index

S

T

V

W

Z

About the Authors

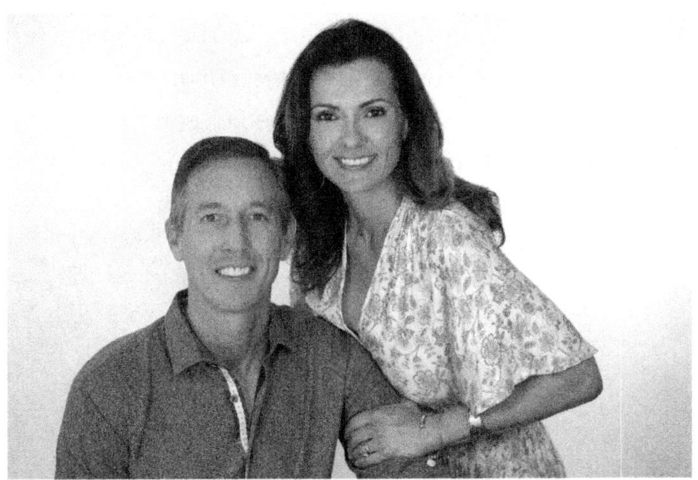

ANA-MARIA TEMPLE, MD

Ana-Maria Temple, MD, has been practicing medicine since 1995 and has treated more than 38,000 patients. She currently lives in Charlotte, NC, with her husband and three children. Her practice, Integrative Health Carolinas, has successfully helped hundreds of moms transform their children's skin with fewer medications. In her mission to change 10,000 families' lives this year, she has created an online Eczema Transformation Program. A regular guest on national news broadcasts and numerous health and wellness podcasts, she continuously educates parents on various social media platforms.

JOHN TEMPLE, MD

John Temple, MD, is a board-certified Orthopedic Surgeon who practiced for over twenty years before leaving to pursue holistic medicine. Once he realized that making a lifestyle change and getting to the root cause of disease was a better long-term approach to health than surgical measures, he made it his mission to educate the public on chronic disease in children, along with his wife, Dr. Ana-Maria Temple. The Temples currently reside in Charlotte, NC, with their three children and their loyal dog. John Temple now builds online health courses focusing on childhood disease. He has launched an online supplement store and writes a wellness blog at DrAnaMaria.com.

Printed in Great Britain
by Amazon

35628227R00145